Robert A. Roush, PhD

Complementary and Alternative Medicine
Clinic Design

More pre-publication
REVIEWS, COMMENTARIES, EVALUATIONS . . .

"This book offers hope. Encouraging the integration of CAM with traditional medicine, the author strongly urges clients' self-awareness and choice. He places both the patient and the doctor in the driver's seat when developing a health care plan. The author challenges patients to know themselves, seek what they need, and realize that their beliefs and choices can positively impact their health and sense of well-being. A good read for anyone interested in holistic care and delivery."

Reverend Nancy Adams, MDiv
United Church of Christ Clergywoman;
Board Certified Chaplain in Association
of Professional Chaplains;
Chaplain at St. Luke's Hospital,
Bethlehem, PA

"*Complementary and Alternative Medicine* is a unique and comprehensive review of complementary medicine. Dr. Roush's approach of bringing CAM together with conventional medicine in a clinical setting is just the prescription for today's ailing health care system."

Ken Levin, MD
Medical Director,
College Heights Imaging,
Allentown, PA

The Haworth Integrative Healing Press®
An Imprint of The Haworth Press, Inc.
New York • London • Oxford

Complementary and Alternative Medicine
Clinic Design

THE HAWORTH INTEGRATIVE HEALING PRESS
Ethan Russo
Editor

The Last Sorcerer: Echoes of the Rainforest by Ethan Russo

Professionalism and Ethics in Complementary and Alternative Medicine by John Crellin and Fernando Ania

Cannabis and Cannabinoids: Pharmacology, Toxicology, and Therapeutic Potential by Franjo Grotenhermen and Ethan Russo

Modern Psychology and Ancient Wisdom: Psychological Healing Practices from the World's Religious Traditions edited by Sharon G. Mijares

Complementary and Alternative Medicine: Clinic Design by Robert A. Roush

Complementary and Alternative Medicine
Clinic Design

Robert A. Roush, PhD

The Haworth Integrative Healing Press®
An Imprint of The Haworth Press, Inc.
New York • London • Oxford

Published by

The Haworth Integrative Healing Press®, an imprint of The Haworth Press, Inc., 10 Alice Street, Binghamton, NY 13904-1580.

PUBLISHER'S NOTE
This book should not be used as a substitute for treatment by a professional health care provider. The reader should consult a physician for matters relating to symptoms that may require medical attention.

Cover design by Jennifer M. Gaska.

Cover graphic representing the chakra divisions by Steven H. Olofson.

Library of Congress Cataloging-in-Publication Data

Roush, Robert A.
    Complementary and alternative medicine : clinic design / Robert A. Roush.
        p. cm.
    Includes bibliographical references and index.
    ISBN 0-7890-1803-9 (alk. paper) — ISBN 0-7890-1804-7 (soft)
    1. Alternative medicine. I. Title.

R733 .R677 2003
615.5—dc21

                                        2002068772

CONTENTS

ABOUT THE AUTHOR

Robert Roush received his PhD in Complementary and Alternative Health from Westbrook University in Aztec, New Mexico. He holds a certificate in Ayurvedic healing from the American Institute of Vedic Studies in Santa Fe, New Mexico, and is an adjunct professor of Yoga and Meditation, Northampton Community College, Bethlehem, Pennsylvania.

In 1978, Dr. Roush began his career in nonprofit health services, co-founding the Western New York Alzheimer's Disease Association. The following year, he presented research findings on the neurotransmitter acetylcholine and nutrition at Millard Fillmore Hospital in Buffalo, New York. After receiving his master's degree in nonprofit administration in 1988, he was named Division Director of the American Heart Association of Southwestern New York in Jamestown, where he administered programs including education on lifestyles training for school-aged children and physician offices, community, food, cooking, nutrition, and exercise programs, and emergency cardiac programs.

In 1991, Dr. Roush was named Executive Director of the AIDS Services Center in Bethlehem, Pennsylvania, where he studied immunology as related to the HIV virus and started a resource library of nutritional, herbal, and alternative therapies including humor therapy and the spiritual aspects of health care. The center offered the medical community a continuing education program in complementary and alternative therapies for HIV/AIDS. Currently, Dr. Roush is Clinical Director (and Co-Founder) of the 7 Senses Health Center in Bethlehem.

Preface

With hospitals, private clinics, and individual practices establishing complementary and alternative medicine (CAM) programs, guidelines and standards need to be established.

It is important to note here that these guidelines, which will present consistency and create a basis for quality, are not created to protect the public from itself or from "quacks" who seek to take advantage of incurable disease states. First, there will always be those who seek to take advantage of people regardless of any guidelines, standards, or licensing laws. Licensing laws were originally intended to set standards and restrictions concerning the practice of health care, rather than protect patients. Civil laws about causing harm to others and committing fraud are the laws that protect the public (Wilson, 1998). Recently, licensing has sought to lighten the burden on the public for such litigation, and many local and discipline-based organizations and boards in medicine have truly sought to assure quality. However, this has not reduced the litigious tendency of the public toward medicine. Indeed, such litigation is rampant. Second, the public is now far more educated than given credit. It is almost shockingly unprecedented to suggest that people may be able to get enough information and be intelligent enough to make their own decisions about health care, but this is the model of holism and of CAM: partnerships with patients in which patients make the decisions. Last, and especially in the United States, the public will decide what health care it will consume, where it will consume it, and when. The precepts of a consumer society have prevailed in our culture and, for better or worse, health care must now fit this model to survive. Through the study and application of successful clinical models drawing from medicine, psychology, and social services, an effective model for a clinic can be established that refines and uses holism.

Such a model contends that mind, body, and spirit are considered in each condition of human health and disease. Emerging and traditional techniques (i.e., Ayurveda, Chinese medicine, Reiki, reflexology, prayer, homeopathy, massage) are herein analyzed for effectiveness in the context of five simple domains or classifications: alternative medical systems, mind/body interventions, biologically based interventions, body-based manipulation therapies, and energy/metaphysical therapies. These techniques do not stand alone, but rather complement one another. It is also recommended that these modalities be integrated with current medical care, and that conventional medicine recognize when another modality may indeed have a better, or at least a less harmful, way.

Education for practitioners of these modalities is discussed. Standards for quality and an approach for creating "accreditation" are addressed, as well as clarification of accreditation and how it can be applied to disparate modalities.

How a clinic or combined practice can be structured is addressed. The political structure of medicine in general and the political structure of organizations such as clinics and hospitals have dramatically impacted the health of those consuming care. These questions must also be considered to create a successful model for health care.

I once watched a television episode of *60 Minutes* about complementary and alternative medicine with Ed Bradley interviewing Andrew Weil, MD. Dr. Arnold Seymour Relman, MD, one of Andrew Weil's former college professors at Harvard University, was complaining that Dr. Weil gave people false hope and that the scientific evidence Dr. Weil used for his claims about alternative medicine was "flimsy." Dr. Relman was quoted as saying, "What I take Andy to task for is that he allows people to believe that very often you can cure these serious physical ailments by belief and mysticism . . . There's not a shred of evidence that it's so." If one has actually read Dr. Weil's books, he often does discuss the role of belief in illness and recovery, and he does so in the context of medicine, CAM modalities, and good, old-fashioned, pure research. From the beginning, the "camps" of "expert" against "nut-case" were established by the report.

The most interesting tool used in the report was the image-play of how Dr. Relman appeared (a kind face and wearing a suit as the established Harvard doctor) versus how Dr. Weil appeared (mostly shown in ethnic-style clothing, sitting in a meditation position, or up-close with his odd, puffy beard). It was implied that Dr. Weil was some kind of whacked weirdo. With the use of the American cultural 1950s' image of conservatism in Dr. Relman, what the report was really saying was, "Gosh, Beaver, how can you believe a guy like Andy Weil? He's not like us . . . let's stay away from and be afraid of what we don't understand."

Of course, commentator Ed Bradley seemed to be on the side of the conventional wisdom of conventional medicine, and joined in the implication that Dr. Weil is a con artist. What was entirely absent from the report was the idea of *complementary* medicine. Commentator Morley Safer dramatically told the audience at the end of the segment that an interviewee who used breathing and meditation to help with cancer had "had a relapse and was now taking chemotherapy." I doubt that this patient had ever abandoned his conventional treatment, but rather had *enhanced* his health and sense of well-being through complementary medicine. This patient stated that his quality of life and his hope had inexorably been altered by his experience with CAM.

Have we moved to the need for lab indicators or scientific evidence to tell us how we *feel* at any given time? The human immune system has been functioning just fine for millennia, and it has done so before anyone had the slightest *scientific* idea of how it works, thank you very much.

Mr. Bradley's news account then proceeded to tell us that the products Dr. Weil recommends contain fewer active ingredients than their labels indicate. I wonder: How can something have an "active ingredient" when it is implied that the ingredient is "mystical" and no evidence exists that it works? As for flimsy evidence regarding efficacy, the segment failed to refer to questionable drug-trial reports that provided the basis for conventional medications' approval in the United States, or recent reports that medications such as Claritin and Proventil, contain neither sufficient quantities of listed ingredients nor any of the "active ingredient."

What Dr. Relman was undoubtedly referring to was Dr. Weil's belief that the "placebo effect" is a power that should be harnessed. Dr. Relman knows that approximately one-third of persons taking a placebo seem to get better, skewing the results of drug trials and having to be compensated for. Since only approximately 10 percent of individuals seem to spontaneously recover from illness (with no treatment), the placebo effect is a very real conundrum.

The need for more research concerning how to use complementary and alternative medicine modalities together with conventional medicine became evident during the research I conducted for this book. The patient clearly knows that these CAM methods make her or him *feel better.* The idea that *how we feel* must wait for verification from the lab or approval from a physician is one of the main problems that has driven patients away from what we now call conventional medicine. Ironically, as Division Director of an American Heart Association office in southwestern New York, and as Executive Director of an AIDS center in Bethlehem, Pennsylvania, I have repeatedly seen the power of lab tests in causing a more rapid *deterioration* of the health of patients, and I am certain it has caused more rapid deaths. Although I conducted no study to prove the correlation of these assertions, I need no study to prove that these patients all *felt worse.* Their rapid onset of symptoms and deterioration subsequent to negative lab indicators are also part of their client records.

None of the health techniques described herein are brand new. Some are as old, and even older, than the tradition that brought us the American Medical Association (AMA) in the United States. These CAM modalities are now just raising their heads; are gaining authority; and are being considered on par with, or along with, more commonly asserted methods. This has to do with so many factors, that the occasional news report crying "charlatanry" will have little to no effect.

This book then, is dedicated to the day when no more "camps" in health care will exist—when the type of treatment offered will have more to do with the individual's health than promoting any one particular brand of medicine, or any one person's or group's view of good health.

Chapter 1

Review of Complementary and Alternative Modalities

This work uses a modification of the five domains created by the National Institutes of Health's Office of Complementary and Alternative Medicine (CAM). CAM practitioners from around the United States worked with government officials and other medical personnel to create these classifications during the Clinton administration. These original classifications or domains have been slightly modified here to enable them to incorporate education, licensing, and regulation needs for CAM. Specifically, some "energy" therapies have been moved to the "biologically based" classification, including magnetic therapy, since magnetic fields are both detectable and measurable, and their effects can be measured in reasonable randomized trials overseen by the Food and Drug Administration (FDA). The "Energy" domain has been updated to include "Metaphysical" as part of the title. This energy/metaphysical domain removes prayer from the mind/body category as an "undetectable" (at least not detectable without much argument) means of intervention: prayer asks an outside, metaphysical force to intervene. The energy/metaphysical category now includes Reiki, shamanism, and therapeutic touch, not due to a lack of conventional scientific proof but because it will be recommended here that licensing and regulation for such modalities be classified in the same way that religious and faith-based means of intervention have always been classified, and that is to be exempt from such constraints.

The modalities discussed in this chapter are by no means exhaustive. This underscores one of the public problems with CAM—so many new interventions seem to appear every day. Despite the possibility that some of these interventions might become established as highly effective for the treatment of various conditions, this flux of modalities adds to the appearance of faddishness of CAM to both consumers and current health professionals. Where the expression "drug of the week" refers to the rapid development and release of new medications in the United States, so does a CAM "modality of the week" reflect this proliferation of new methods. This is more likely due to the nature of our "try and discard" culture than to anything good for health care. It would therefore be useful to adopt a five-domain classification system, so one can quickly refer to a modality as falling within an easily understood classification or type.

Part of the purpose of this chapter is to offer some information about scientific studies done for CAM modalities to assist prospective clinics in choosing which modalities to offer. Something must be said here about what this "scientific proof" of efficacy is. The double-blind, placebo-controlled study for pharmaceutical drugs has been entrenched in the United States since 1962. Since that time, this method has been exalted as the only true scientific method by which all medical research must now be conducted. It is hard to believe that no amount of clinical evidence or other forms of scientific evidence will suffice for this "true and ultimate scientific method." The author has heard the lament and cry of dozens of practitioners concerning the difficulty of developing a placebo for such things as massage so that we will never even know if it is effective! This reasoning is faulty. The method and FDA regulation set forth in 1962 was put into place to determine whether drugs were safe and effective. If a method is safe, it does not need scrutiny in this regard, unless one touts that doing anything at all is "unsafe." For this view, the author sighs and places his face in his hands. If living is unsafe, the solution for you is alarming because it involves not living.

The "effective" part of the equation has become dependent on the placebo variable, because it has been defined to mean "more effective than placebo." The whole "placebo effect" was defined when it was discovered that persons given something—anything that they thought was a cure—got better whether or not it contained an intended active pharmacological agent. Here it is in frightening nonscientific terms: compared to a control group with no treatment, a sham, or nonsense treatment, is effective for about one-third of persons suffering from clinically verifiable illness. Now, here is a vast curiosity: the same "scientific" persons who know full well that this placebo effect exists, and use it to "prove" that CAM interventions are fanciful ideas that do not work, also purport that no scientific evidence proves a mind/body connection, and that, therefore, mind/body interventions cannot work. This is a curious paradox. This placebo effect is further discussed in the Ayurveda section that follows.

For this placebo question, researchers now compare many CAM practices to drugs that have already been proven more effective than placebo. If a CAM procedure, then, shows equal or better results, it can be proclaimed effective. In the same vein, long-term clinical evidence and observational studies can be used to determine some level of efficacy. Although testimonials do not prove efficacy and may merely show a "placebo of choice" for a patient, it must be asked, "If that procedure is safe and effective for that person, what is the problem?" As long as people understand that "miracle cures" do not exist, and provided CAM clinics do not mislead people into believing in such cures, it may be both reasonable and ethical to offer services that do not have a single shred of "scientific proof."

ALTERNATIVE MEDICAL SYSTEMS

The first domain in the classification structure is alternative medical systems. This domain is the broadest in scope. In other cultures, the conventional Western medical system would be classified within it. It is the most confusing category, as it may include some or all of the elements of other domains. The single most important factor for inclusion in the alternative medical systems domain is a method for assessment of health and diagnosis of disease. A health care system is not a "system" without a concisely developed method for assessment and diagnosis.

This classification is first because it recognizes that health care is primarily a cultural phenomenon, shrouded in the mists of an elongated history that stretches to a time before record keeping. Western medicine has similar deep roots as well. It did not start suddenly when the concept of the Western scientific method was introduced, and it still contains components that predate this type of validation (see Figure 1.1 and 1.2). Health care itself is much older than this. These instincts to survive and care for one another are seen in other species as well, and the ancestors of our own species likely established interdependent helping roles to perform in their social structure. Helping others survive and be well likely would have been cru-

Music & Art

10,000 BC	4000 BC	3000 BC	1200 BC	500 BC	0	500	1000	2000
Rock Painting	Functional objects embellished (first bowls, utensils, then clothes and jewelry)			Architecture becomes prevalent; sculpture, painting, manuscript writing			Medieval art Cathedrals Renaissance	

Commerce

10,000 BC	4000 BC	3000 BC	1200 BC	500 BC	0	500	1000	2000
Hunting and Agriculture	Farms, Domestication	Mercantilism	Roads				The New world and imperialism American capitalism	

Politics

10,000 BC	4000 BC	3000 BC	1200 BC	500 BC	0	500	1000	2000
Family ⟶ Tribe	City-states Unification War	Nations arise Ethnic identity	China enters Golden Era	Ancient Greece	Rome	Dark Ages begin	Charlemagne Age of Conquest	

Religion

10,000 BC	4000 BC	3000 BC	1200 BC	500 BC	0	500	1000	2000
	Fertility: Goddess, Fertilization: God Judaic: Adam and Eve	Egyptian Book of the Dead	Moses Judaic: Abraham	Buddha, Philosophy	Christ	Islam		Pluralism Cultism

Science

10,000 BC	4000 BC	3000 BC	1200 BC	500 BC	0	500	1000	2000
	The wheel	The plough Bronze Age	Food preservation		The abacus The Iron Age		Technology for conquest and commerce—sailing, killing, agriculture	Microscopic Age Atomic Age

Health Care

10,000 BC	4000 BC	3000 BC	1200 BC	500 BC	0	500	1000	2000
The woman as healer: Mother Roots of nutrition and herbology	The woman as healer: Medicine woman The man as healer: Shamanism	Ayurvedic and Chinese medicine Herbology and nutrition come of age			Hippocrates: Roots of Heroic Medicine War Medicine and Surgery come of age			Homeopathy Modern Medicine (allopathic) Osteopathy Chiropractic etc.

FIGURE 1.1. The history of health care graphically shown with overlapping occurrences in science, religion, politics, commerce, and music/art.

FIGURE 1.2. The advent of science and politics in medicine from 1700 to the present, two very important themes in this book. The political history of medicine helps us to understand why we think the way we do about certain types of health care.

	1700	1800	1810	1828	1836	1860	1880	1900	1920	1940	1950	1960	1980	2000
Medicine Types	The Age of Heroic Medicine, leeches, bleeding, noxious drugs	Dr. Hahnemann writes homeopathy treatise in Germany		First homeopathic physician arrives in the U.S.	1835—Allentown Academy—first homeopathic medical school in U.S.	Traditional MDs introduce narcotics	1874—Andrew Taylor Still starts osteopathy; 1866—Mary Baker Eddy starts Christian Science	1896—Dr. Benedict Lust starts naturopathy; 1895—Daniel David Palmer starts chiropractic		Medical schools reorganize to basic chemistry		1962—FDA says drugs must be proven; Dissension among naturopaths	Double-blind drug studies introduced	
The Politics of Medicine and other Politics		1772—Traditional MDs organize and get political clout in U.S. licensing. Leads to popular health movement.			1840—Popular health movement effectively wipes out licensing to make way for homeopathic practice. Women active politically. Prevention introduced.	1846—AMA organizes to fight popularists. Homeopaths excluded as practitioners of "exclusive dogma." War ensues.	AMA takes over local health and hospital boards, refuses to admit women, and aggressively hounds homeopaths. The popular health movement dissolves. / 1865—Civil War. Lincoln orders tissue samples. More soldiers die of influenza than battle wounds. Clara Barton is on the battlefield.	Homeopaths and allopaths unite briefly to oppose licensing of osteopaths. / 1881—Clara Barton founds the Red Cross.						
							WOMEN'S SUFFRAGE ———————		—— WOMEN WIN VOTE					
Science	Microscopes become important, but are not extremely powerful		Telegraph	Photography		Modern scientific method becomes universal	1885—Louis Pasteur and rabies vaccine discovered; 1895—X-rays discovered	Physics introduces quantum theory; Einstein's influence on science begins; Microscope becomes powerful	1929—penicillin discovered; 1941—penicillin used effectively			Electron microscope refined; DNA discovered		

5

cial roles played by individuals for the survival of the entire group. The ill health of wise leaders or skilled workers before their apprentices could learn these skills might have led to great suffering and death for many members of the group. Health care, therefore, became a necessity for the ancestors of our species. This role of health care provider, in most instances, was and still is performed by the head female or mother of the family unit. This intimate form of health care has a sustained prevalence in many cultures throughout the world and should not be taken lightly.

A dramatic example of this intimate health care appeared in the alumni newsletter of Jefferson Medical College, Philadelphia, Pennsylvania. It reported that William Fair, a renowned cancer surgeon, was diagnosed with a colon tumor. After two surgeries and a year of chemotherapy the cancer continued. No progress ensued until his wife Mary Ann insisted that he try an alternative approach: meditation, yoga, a change in diet, and Chinese herbs led the tumor to shrink. Fair claims he scientifically evaluated his options when selecting his alternative treatments, and now he lectures about the use of complementary and alternative therapies, but it was his wife's role as their family health care manager that led him in the right direction, despite his own expertise and experience in the field (Clendenin, 2000).

At the time health care began to organize as a recognizable discipline, civilization itself was emerging from familial and tribal forms of social structure. The dynamics of cooperation and oppression coalesced in order to create improved and enhanced living conditions, in order to bend the will of the many to the will of the few. Clashes occurred and wars were declared; this dynamic struggle to fight and to tend to the wounded is inexorably attached to the advancement and knowledge of organized health care.

The advent of religion and the pursuit of thought in an organized manner in the ancient cultures of India, China, and Greece led to the creation or formalization of the nurturing, or feminine, form of health care. The scientific method of observing and reflecting on thousands of health cases, along with what were essentially trial-and-error treatment methods, were drawn together with meditative thought in ancient India. Causes and effects were observed and recorded. An entire scientific explanation for the construct of the universe was created and written down in the ancient Indian Vedas, the earliest Hindu sacred writings. Buddhists also played important roles in recording these observations, including the effort of the first Dalai Lama who called physicians from both China and India to systematically record their knowledge, thus creating the Tibetan medicine system. In Greece, it was the same, with great observers of nature and philosophers such as Hippocrates giving the first formalized direction in health care in the West.

Chinese Medicine

As one of the oldest and most detailed systems of health care, Chinese medicine has recently returned to some prominence in Western cultures because one of its components, acupuncture, has had considerable success in meeting current randomized-trial standards for efficacy. For the purposes of reviewing the literature here, meta-analyses have been used whenever possible. Meta-analyses of studies about the effects of acupuncture on pain show positive differences between acupuncture and no intervention, and equal results between acupuncture and other therapies (Melchart et al., 1999; Ernst and White, 1998; Riet, Kleijnen, and Knipschild, 1990; Patel et al., 1989). However, the use of placebo or "sham acupuncture" continues to present a problem in these studies. Most of the meta-analyses authors suggested caution and warned about what they felt were poorly constructed studies. Acupuncture was catapulted into the forefront of CAM modalities in 1997 when *The New York Times,* on November 6, published it as front-page news (Weil, 1997a). The original press release from the National Institutes of Health (NIH) stated,

> A consensus panel convened by the National Institutes of Health (NIH) today concluded there is clear evidence that needle acupuncture treatment is effective for postoperative and chemotherapy nausea and vomiting, nausea of pregnancy, and postoperative dental pain. The twelve-member panel also concluded in their consensus statement that there are a number of other pain-related conditions for which acupuncture may be effective as an adjunct therapy, an acceptable alternative, or as part of a comprehensive treatment program but for which there is less convincing scientific data. These conditions include but are not limited to addiction, stroke rehabilitation, headache, menstrual cramps, tennis elbow, fibromyalgia (general muscle

pain), low back pain, carpal tunnel syndrome, and asthma. (NIH, 1997)

This consensus panel derived its observations from what it felt were several good single studies. After this time, the AMA started reporting the research in earnest and the *Journal of the American Medical Association (JAMA)* began to brim full with positive acupuncture results. An online index for *JAMA* listed 176 articles published from 1997 to 2001, most of them quite favorable (*JAMA*, 2001). The odd thing is that positive results were scant for acupuncture before this time. This may illustrate an important point about politics and science: the panel was a political body, which issued an opinion based on unquoted sources. Since the panel was U.S. government sponsored, its opinion entrenched itself in public opinion (especially since it was reported in *The New York Times*) and was picked up by the prestigious AMA. This may also indicate an important factor in the effectiveness of any health modality: cultural acceptance.

Ayurveda

Between 3,000 and 6,000 years ago, the Indian Vedas were established, first as an oral tradition and then as sacred writings, ushering in this health care system of India (Frawley, 1989). Since this is the author's base discipline, it should not be construed that in-depth observations in this section are exclusive to Ayurveda, or that other systems of health care do not have methodologies and insights as effective or more effective than that of Ayurveda.

Ayur is the Sanskrit word for "life," and *veda* the word for "science." It can also be translated as the "study of longevity." This is important to understanding the purpose of Ayurvedic intervention and prescriptions: to prolong life in order to pursue spiritual goals. This clearly ranks the importance of the "holistic trinity" of mind, body, and spirit—something that most religious or spiritual traditions might agree with, but that most health practices do not cover. This is, however, inseparable from the Ayurvedic view.

It is difficult to locate studies on panchakarma, the main Ayurvedic therapeutic technique that focuses on using the body's natural systems of elimination to cleanse and detoxify. Since Ayurveda is heavily lifestyle oriented, most of the interest in this modality has focused on diet and herbs, with those interested in metaphysical or "new age" ideals, focusing on color and gem therapy, as well as chakra balancing (Chakras are metaphysical energy crossroads where the nadis—similar to the Chinese meridians—intersect. These energy centers, when balanced, are considered to affect physical organs, emotional and mental states, and spiritual development.) and the more spiritual aspects of the discipline. The U.S. National Library of Medicine available via their Web site, Medline, contains the most significant studies.

In review of all these alternative medical systems, a question arises: Should Western consumers afford the same respect to the medical systems of other cultures as they do their own? (This is a double-edged sword! U.S. citizens, especially, are sharply critical of their medical care.) It seems clear that only simple arrogance would discount the scientific methods followed by another culture, even if those methods do not match those of our own. The question of scientific method as required by federal authorities—such as in drug approval—is a study unto itself. Many criticisms of CAM assert that it should have to hold up to the same scientific rigor as other medical treatments (Council on Scientific Affairs, 2001) and yet it is little understood that the whole process of drug trials is a relatively recent U.S. phenomenon from the 1960s, which is not as well managed as it is touted as being (Weil, 1995, 1980). The placebo effect in drug trials has never been well accounted for. The fact that a sugar-containing pill is used for comparison purposes (as sugar has a specific metabolic effect and chemical structure) is, perhaps, one of the most fundamental mistakes of this method.

The rigors of Ayurveda for effectiveness in its own structure as a science rely on the one common element of science regardless of culture, which is *observation.* However, Ayurvedic observation is a passive activity (Frawley, 1989). Ayurveda as a science does not allow for the introduction of theory into observation—at least not beyond the concept that one is going to try out an idea. Hypotheses for results are quite strictly forbidden. In addition, a meditative state must be achieved by the observer, so that such things as hypotheses can be kept at bay while the observed subject reveals its true nature to the scientist. In other words, through formal tradition and training in mind-discipline techniques such as meditation, Ayurveda as a science has a means for eliminating bias. It also stands to reason that a health care system with clinical application ranging in thousands of years has a basis in science. There would have to be some efficacy and safety in most of the methods, or it would not be so widely accepted by that culture. As for who is a "magician" mumbling incantations of gibberish over the bodies of the afflicted, try rattling the pages of a *JAMA* article declaring line after line of "P values" for cancer lab indicators over the body of a dying patient. One may as well: the fact is, no method has all the answers and the sooner the modalities work together, rather than questioning one another's integrity, the sooner we will reach a world medicine that will offer the most options for wellness to all patients.

Today in India, a strong movement of Western-trained scientists is looking at the traditional Ayurvedic herbs and herb compounds, verifying their efficacy, and isolating the active component in conventional Western pharmaceutical style. Western-style studies have also verified the effectiveness of some subtleties of Ayurvedic treatment, such as the use of palliative treatment alone, or with cleansing treatment (Nagashayana et al., 2000) for Parkinson's disease. This study showed that the complete set of panchakarma techniques when administered together is more effective than palliative treatment alone. This is important news, because it may suggest that treatments that are common in many types of medicine can be made more effective if an Ayurvedic regimen is introduced.

Eighty-one studies focusing on multiple areas of Ayurveda were found in a Medline Internet search on Ayurveda. Thirty-three studies were usable as lab experiments (see Table 1.1). Only two studies showed results contrary to Ayurvedic practice. The contrary studies were general commentaries on Ayurveda, or inconclusive, according to the authors. Twenty-five of the studies were for pharmaceutical agents that were compared to Western drugs and had been shown to be as effective or more effective. Only one study was a meta-analysis (Lodha and Bagga, 2000), which, without surprise, concluded that more, higher quality studies needed to be done. Although one study used a control group receiving no treatment ("An Alternative Medicine Treatment for Parkinson's Disease," 1995), none of the studies used the double-blind procedure. In fact, most of these studies were either in vitro or animal studies. These studies reveal a very strong, if not overwhelming, need to create double-blind trials of Ayurvedic compounds for efficacy.

TABLE 1.1. Summary of Thirty-One Studies of Ayurveda

Journal	First Author		Title	Results	Year
Arzneimittelfor-schung	Arjungi	KN	Areca nut: A review	The ingredient in betel nut that causes cancer	1976
Journal of Ethnopharmacology	Atal	CK	Scientific evidence on the role of Ayurvedic herbals on bioavailability of drugs	Presumably human study on digest aid trikatu effectively increasing bioavailability of drugs	1981
Social Science & Medicine	Weiss	DR	Traditional concepts of mental disorder among Indian psychiatric patients: preliminary report of work in progress	Ayurvedic patients seeking allopathic mental health care due to ineffectiveness of Ayurveda	1986
Prostaglandins Leukot Essential Fatty Acids	Srivastava	KC	Extracts from two frequently consumed spices—cumin *(Cuminum cyminum)* and turmeric *(Curcuma longa)*—inhibit platelet aggregation and alter eicosanoid biosynthesis in human blood platelets	Effective in vitro anti-inflammatory action of cumin	1989
Journal of Ethnopharmacology	Saraf	MN	Studies on the mechanism of action of *Semecarpus anacardium* in rheumatoid arthritis	Animal study arthritic treatment, lab indicators, shows effectiveness	1989
Journal of Post-graduate Medicine	Dalvi	SS	Effect of *Asparagus racemosus* (Shatavari) on gastric emptying time in normal healthy volunteers	Favorable comparison to Western drugs, Shatavari as a laxative	1990
Prostaglandins Leukot Essential Fatty Acids	Smith	DE	Selective growth inhibition of a human malignant melanoma cell line by sesame oil in vitro	Effective lab in vitro control of cancer cells by sesame seed oil	1992
Indian Journal of Experimental Biology	Alam	M	Anti-inflammatory and antipyretic activity of vicolides of *Vicoa indica* DC	Animal study showed potent anti-inflammatory in liver and blood lab indicators	1992
Journal of Ethnopharmacology	Ramanujam	S	Amrita bindu—a salt-spice-herbal health food supplement for the prevention of ·nitrosamine induced depletion of antioxidants	Human trial of Amrita Bindu, reversing artificially induced antioxidant loss as detected in liver and blood cells	1994
Journal of Alternative and Complementary Medicine	Journal editorial		An alternative medicine treatment for Parkinson's disease: Results of a multi-center clinical trial	Favorable comparison to Western Levadopa and a control group for Parkinson's	1995
Journal of Ethnopharmacology	Labadie	RP	Ayurvedic herbal drugs with possible cytostatic activity	Ayurvedic herbs decrease tumor cell growth in vitro	1995

TABLE 1.1 *(continued)*

Journal	First Author		Title	Results	Year
Prostaglandins Leukot Essential Fatty Acids	Srivastava	KC	Curcumin, a major component of food spice turmeric *(Curcuma longa)* inhibits aggregation and alters eicosanoid metabolism in human blood platelets	Curcumin lab indicators as an anti-inflammatory	1995
HPB Surgery	Thorat	SP	Emblica officinalis: A novel therapy for acute pancreatitis—an experimental study	Animal study anti-inflammatory, shows effectiveness	1995
Indian Journal of Experimental Biology	Agnihotri	S	A novel approach to study antibacterial properties of volatile components of selected Indian medicinal herbs	Shows aroma molecules kill bacteria	1996
Journal of Postgraduate Medicine	Tamhane	MD	Effect of oral administration of *Terminalia chebula* on gastric emptying: An experimental study	Animal study laxative, shown effective	1997
Indian Journal of Experimental Biology	Singh	RK	Pharmacological actions of *Pongamia pinnata* roots in albino rats	Animal study antiulcer, shows effectiveness	1997
Journal of Alternative and Complementary Medicine	Bhattacharya	SK	Effect of trasina, an Ayurvedic herbal formulation, on experimental models of Alzheimer's disease and central cholinergic markers in rats	Animal study reversed artificially induced memory loss in rats	1997
Cancer Lett	Bhide	SV	Effect of turmeric oil and turmeric oleoresin on cytogenetic damage in patients suffering from oral submucous fibrosis	Lab indicators for turmeric as anti-inflammatory	1997
Medicine Care Research and Review	Misra	R	Modern drug development from traditional medicinal plants using radioligand receptor-binding assays	Herbal extracts show biological activity	1998
Indian Journal of Medical Research	Bajaj	S	Analgesic activity of gold preparations used in Ayurveda and Unani-Tibb	Animal study analgesic, shows effectiveness	1998
Indian Journal of Experimental Biology	Singh	RK	Pharmacological actions of Abies pindrow Royle leaf	Animal study anti-inflammatory, antiulcer, hypnotic barbiturate shows effectiveness	1998
Indian Journal of Medical Research	Bapat	RD	Leech therapy for complicated varicose veins	Leeches for varicose veins shows effectiveness	1998
Environmental Health Perspectives	Dev	S	Ancient-modern concordance in Ayurvedic plants: Some examples	Confirms use and efficacy of drugs from Ayurvedic herbs	1999

Journal	First Author		Title	Results	Year
Australian and New Zealand Journal of Psychiatry	Walter	G	The relevance of herbal treatments for psychiatric practice.	Lab indicators for intestinal regulation	1999
Indian Journal of Experimental Biology	Bhattacharya	SK	Adaptogenic activity of Siotone, a polyherbal formulation of Ayurvedic rasayanas	Favorable comparison to Western pharmaceuticals	2000
Phytomedicine	Bhattacharya	SK	Anxiolytic-antidepressant activity of *Withania somnifera* glycowithanolides: An experimental study	Favorable comparison to Western pharmaceuticals	2000
Phytotherapy Research	Bhattacharya	A	Effect of *Withania somnifera* glycowithanolides on iron-induced hepatotoxicity in rats	Establishes active ingredient	2000
Indian Journal of Experimental Biology	Patil	S	Antianaemic properties of ayurvedic drugs, raktavardhak, punarnavasav, and navayas louh in albino rats during phenylhydrazine-induced haemolytic anaemia	Shows mechanism of cure	2000
Annals of Academic Medicine Singapore	Lohda	R	Traditional Indian systems of medicine	Concludes more high-quality studies need to be done	2000
Phytotherapy Research	Singh	RK	Pharmacological activity of *Elaeocarpus sphaericus*	Animal study anti-inflammatory, shown effective	2000
Phytotherapy Research	Pohocha	N	Antispasmodic activity of the fruits of *Helicteres isora* Linn.	Favorable comparison to Western pharmaceuticals	2001

From a holistic perspective, it is interesting to note that only three of the studies compared an herb or aroma for efficacy. All the rest compared pharmaceutical derivations of an "active ingredient," as in Western pharmacology. Although the two herb and one aroma studies showed efficacy, other commentary articles did not address this issue, but instead addressed the issue that health decisions were being made from the results of in vitro and animal studies: the same complaints which eventually led to the U.S. FDA rules for safety and efficacy.

Tibetan Medicine

A look at Eastern medical systems would be incomplete without looking at Tibetan medicine, which in and of itself is a derivative system. The current interest in how to integrate health modalities for the benefit of all is not the first time the world has been through such a struggle. In seventh- to eighth-century Tibet, the Dalai Lama had the interest (and apparently the authority) to call physicians together from the medical systems of the geographical areas of what are now China, Persia, India, and Greece in order to study their health systems (Tokar, 1998). Although these systems were found markedly different, they were also found complementary. By the eleventh century, the meticulous recordings of Buddhist monks realized the most complete written system of medical care in history. The government of Tibet in exile still runs the medical school of Tibet, now located in North India. It has a rigorous seven-year curriculum.

Homeopathy

Developed by German physician Samuel Hahnemann in Europe of the early 1800s, homeopathy contends that the minute, trace, or even the *former* minute or trace presence of a substance in a solution can bring about a cure or healing response. It is based on the theory that the treatment substance used must actually cause the same *symptoms* as the disease and that its administration stimulates the body's own healing response.

Homeopathy is a Western-based science with a vast materia medica and a large body of empirical evidence in its volumes of provings (Weil, 1995). It also has one of the most thorough systems (if not the most thorough system) of assessment and diagnosis in Western medicine. This system has been specifically designed to point toward the correct match for treatment. It encompasses not only physical symptoms but also classifies illness into mind/body types that theorize a root cause to chronic illness. Despite a long period of science frowning on homeopathy, it still fills a void for treatment of long-term and troublesome ailments that Western medicine has never come close to addressing. Of interest, after being criticized as a "fanciful treatment based on nonsense," homeopathy leaves less to chance or intuition in its diagnosis procedure than do other medical systems.

Homeopathy remains a curiosity because it still has widespread disagreement as to a theory of its mechanism of action. Such theories that the molecules leave some type of "ghost-like trail" or "impression" in the solution seem to grab at straws more than offer serious possibilities for the true mechanism. Classifying this intervention as an alternative medical system may be a misnomer. As discussed in the energy/metaphysical therapies section, the concept of nonlocal mind may have a solid traditional scientific basis. This theory purports that the *intention* of those preparing the medication may be a required ingredient. Studies showing both the efficacy and inefficacy of homeopathy abound. However, the most careful meta-analyses *do show* that homeopathy is effective in the treatment of many conditions, even in placebo-controlled studies (Ullman, 1991). In fact, evidence supporting homeopathy is quite overwhelming. Oscillococcinum, a substance shown to effectively treat flu and colds, has been studied ad nauseam (Ullman, 1991).

Despite a possible link to intent, effectiveness is also tied to the original or mother substance, and may therefore be due to a misunderstood relationship that a human mind can have with a particular substance at a molecular level. Such a classification still belongs to the metaphysical realm, as it implies currently *undetectable* forces by Western scientific means. It must be cautioned that not accepting a modality because its mechanism is not known or detectable may be discarding a large realm of effective interventions. First, many current treatments accepted in modern medicine are based on unknown action (Weil, 1980) and, second, mechanisms of the cause of disease (such as the detection of bacteria and its observation in the disease process) were at first resisted by the public and scientists alike.

The ire that homeopathy raises in scientific circles must be looked at seriously to bring attention to the political nature of science. A former friend of the author who holds a PhD in chemistry and is employed at a chemical firm emphatically stated that homeopathy could not work because the solution does not contain any of the original molecules of the mother solution. Although he is a chemist who deals with solving problems such as making more-durable epoxies for use in painting bridges, he was perfectly willing to dismiss a form of treatment due to a rudimentary scientific understanding of it. The situation became so emotional that the personal friendship was terminated when the author suggested that perhaps the mechanism for homeopathy was unknown and that it should be used if double-blind studies proved it effective.

A book reviewed in the November 11, 1998, edition of *JAMA, The Alternative Medicine Handbook* (1998) by Barrie R. Cassileth, PhD, is referred to with high regard. The instances of highly positive reviews of scholarship on CAM in *JAMA* are rare. When Cassileth reviews scientific evidence for homeopathy, she states, "Scientifically acceptable proof of homeopathy's effectiveness awaits testing" (Cassileth, 1998, p. 39). Since Dana Ullman had meticulously presented such proof by 1989 in her first edition, and even more conscientiously updated it in 1995, we can assume this information was available to Cassileth, yet it is completely ignored in her work. If it is because Ullman uses British and other studies (as opposed to exclusively U.S. studies), the AMA and its respected authors should consider broadening their literature reviews. Although homeopaths admit the need for more research, the most recent meta-analyses of Oscillococcinum indicate clear statistical significance for its use in reducing the duration of the influenza (Vickers and Smith, 2001).

Such scientific "side taking," despite clear evidence, is not new. In 1988, in a carefully designed study, Dr. Jacques Benveniste (see Ullman, 1991) showed that a homeopathic mixture of antibodies could affect basophils (white blood cells) in vitro. Seventy experiments were run, showing a clear reactivity. This was confirmed by scientists at three other universities. The study drew such widespread disbelief (and ire) that James Randi, the magician, and Walter Stewart, a fraud expert, were called in to debunk the experiment. Randi and Stewart required that a third level of blindness (triple blindness) be added to the experiment. The technician placing the solution on slides was also not to know which solution was placebo. The experiment was run four more times, succeeding once and failing three times; it was instantly decried in such publications as *Time* and *Newsweek* contributing to efforts to debunk homeopathy (Ullman, 1991). What Randi and Stewart may have unwittingly proven is what Larry Dossey, MD, calls "nonlocal mind" (described in the energy/metaphysical section). The third blindness may have removed enough of the intent to make it less effective; the negative intent of the "debunkers" may have affected the substance; or triple blindness may have made them err in tabulating the results. Nonetheless, evidence may now suggest that an interaction occurs between molecules of the mother substance and the intent of those preparing a homeopathic solution. Such an argument points at last to the working mechanism of homeopathy, and is fully within the bounds of physics (see the section on Prayer, Shamanism, and Spirit in Medicine at the end of this chapter).

Naturopathy

Naturopathy can be thought of as a branch of Western medicine that has been practiced but was not named as a discipline until the late nineteenth century. Naturopathy encompasses and utilizes several other systems of medicine and the modalities described herein, and it is based on recognition of the body's innate ability to heal (Keegan, 2001). Similar to homeopathy, and to some extent borrowed from it, a thorough system of assessment is used to determine multiple factors for a person's health status, and then recommendations are made for adjusting lifestyle to maximize health, as well as treatments to address both acute and chronic illness.

Naturopathy has the largest potential to encompass the entire CAM spectrum, and has had a political status similar to osteopathy and chiropractic care, as far as education and licensing go in the United States. Sadly, the discipline has never been organized enough to gain the same foothold that brought accredited education and licensing in all fifty states to the aforementioned disciplines. Naturopathy has floundered with in-fighting, and its organizations have recently lost accreditation recognition by the U.S. Department of Education. A political stronghold of only two naturopathic medical schools has limited the number of accredited schools, thus being unable to produce enough practitioners to compete on par with the other licensed disciplines. As with the past of chiropractic, this has caused the growth of "mail-order diplomas" for naturopathy. Although some of these programs have grown to respectable distance-learning institutions, they remain unaccredited by a body recognized by the U.S. Department of Education. Now, two competing organizations offer testing and credentialing, and most of their energies are spent opposing each other rather than educating the community and becoming the force behind the promotion and successful use of CAM in medical care in the United States today. Traditional Chinese Medicine (TCM) appears to be positioning itself now for this role, as naturopathy loses its influence.

MIND/BODY INTERVENTIONS

The mind/body domain includes traditional Freudian and Jungian psychology as well as techniques from other cultures, similar to the alternative medical systems discussed previously. These particular techniques are focused on the influence of the mind in establishing well-being, and in helping (and being part of) the natural healing process. Techniques such as psychic healing instituted by a person other than the afflicted would not be included in this classification of self-imposed healing.

Societies and cultures have always been fascinated with the power of the mind, and some cultures have created techniques, such as meditation, to harness such power. The expression "mind over matter" is often used as a command to someone suspected of suffering from psychosomatic illness (in other words, a perceived hypochondriac). Some cultures actually consider *all* illness a state of "wrong mind" including that of Ayurveda, which considers illness to be a state of imbalance or "wrong mind" that exists between a person's mind and the consciousness of the universe. Making the proper adjustments in such an imbalance means affecting the cure.

More recently in the United States, Louise Hay in her now classic book *You Can Heal Your Life* (1987), lists, quite exhaustively, various ailments and the psychological root to which they can be ascribed. She describes constipation as, "literally holding on to the same old crap." In other words, constipation is caused by being unable to let go of certain emotionally based problems. This is echoed in Ayurveda, which considers constipation to be a *Vata* (wind) disorder, ruled over by fear. When someone cannot "let go" of a problem, it is usually due to fear. Since all ailments are equated with digestion in Ayurveda, digesting our life experiences and expelling the emotional and psychological waste is just as important as it is in food digestion. Ayurveda does not separate these types of digestion. They are interrelated, and both illustrate a lack of *Pitta,* or "digestive fire." Mind/body techniques seek to find this connection between mental and physical well-being, and prescribe various activities and techniques to be worked from the mental angle.

Yoga

Yoga, the sister science to Ayurveda, has a highly evolved and integrated system for connecting the mind and body. Various techniques for breathing (Pranayama) integrate the connections among autonomic body functions, which can be brought under conscious control. Asanas (the yogic postures) do not merely tone and strengthen muscles, but are aimed at strengthening and toning internal organs and their interrelated systems as well. Slow intense concentration introduces the feel of each muscle group as it moves, and awareness is stimulated. Practitioners relax certain muscles in order to ease into the poses. Most Westerners think yoga ends here, but in fact, this is the very beginning of the introduction to awareness and the mind's control of all bodily functions. Advanced yogis can slow their breathing and even stop the beating of their hearts. Some view this as some type of amazing "circus" act, when it is really a demonstration of the power of mind over matter. For example, concentrating on relaxation and awareness of the location of food in the digestive system can cure and alleviate various digestive disorders.

In a trial for carpal tunnel syndrome reported in *JAMA* (Garfinkle et al., 1998), yoga was found to be more effective than no treatment or wrist splinting in relieving some symptoms and signs of carpal tunnel syndrome. The trial showed that subjects had both increased strength and reduced pain. This study is important because it relates specific yogic techniques to such benefits.

Meditation

Meditation is part of yoga and other healing disciplines, but it is also thought of as being a separate activity. Often, meditation and prayer are misclassified together. The difference is that meditation is personal and internal, whereas prayer is aimed at an external or internal sense of God or spirituality. A good way of considering meditation is as "mind hygiene"—keeping the paths and the channels of the mind open, and allowing the waste to be expelled. In Ayurveda, the mind is considered an organ of no greater importance than the bowels or bladder. The mind, however, processes mental and emotional energies in the forms of images and communications. This makes Ayurvedic psychology strongly divergent from Western psychology. Where Western psychology uses techniques such as psychoanalysis to pinpoint and ascribe deep meaning to emotional events, Ayurveda uses techniques of meditation to clear the debris of such emotional energies. It does not ascribe importance to them any more than a fluid that irritated the bladder is ascribed importance. It is most important to flush the fluid from the bladder so it can heal. Such ideas are not far from Western culture though. In the Rogers and Hammerstein musical *South Pacific,* the main character, Nellie Forbush, declares, "I'm gonna wash that man right outta my hair, and send him on his way!" This is clearly a declaration of cleansing and intended healing for an emotionally unhealthy situation.

Research indicates that meditation is effective in reducing stress and warding off panic. Research at the University of Massachusetts demonstrated a 50 percent reduction in pain for participants in an eight-week program and the American Heart Association found that transcendental meditation (TM) reduced hypertension in the African-American patients participating in a study (Cassileth, 1998).

Biofeedback

Biofeedback is a technique developed in the 1970s that uses equipment to measure physical responses (such as heart rate and blood pressure). These readings are shown to the patient as they occur so that the patient can then find the connection between the mind and body, and consciously slow the heart rate. This technique uses equipment to help realize the same mind/body control that techniques such as yoga or meditation teach.

Art/Music Therapy

Art and music were an important part of therapeutic health techniques in the ancient Greek Asclepions (cliniclike organizations named after Asclepius, the god of healing) (Keegan, 2001). These institutions used the knowledge of the first Western physician, Hippocrates. Drama, music, art, and humor—so important in Greek culture—were used to focus on mental, emotional, and spiritual aspects of illness. Today, art therapies are used to increase expression and therefore to open and clear emotional channels.

Tai Chi Chuan

From about the twelfth century in China, tai chi chuan, commonly called tai chi, is a formal sequence of movements assembled in a flowing way that focuses breathing and awareness in the same way and with some of the same goals as yoga. In addition, self-defense may be a goal of tai chi. Tai chi is linked to Taoism in China, based on the philosophy of "The Way," i.e., balancing the yin and yang principles throughout life. Practicing tai chi builds awareness, and this awareness eventually leads to the same realizations of the power we have in our minds to see how the plane of consciousness precedes and rules over the physical plane.

Tai chi has been shown to enhance cardiopulmonary function in the elderly, as well as in coronary-bypass patients; to relieve chronic back pain; to increase flexibility; and in some studies to lower blood pressure (Keegan, 2001). These results are easily seen as an exercise benefit, and tai chi is therefore a popular part of community fitness programs, hospital cardiac rehab programs, and theater and expressive arts programs.

BIOLOGICALLY BASED INTERVENTIONS

Biologically based interventions are designed to affect the biology of the patients receiving treatment. Pharmaceutical drugs in Western medicine are such an intervention. This classification includes all attempts to influence health by taking any biochemical substance by ingestion, injection, or by other means such as rubbing it on the skin. Here, this category differs from the NIH classification in that it includes any detectable (by current Western scientific means) field or energy as well as biochemical substances, which can include either herbs or nutraceuticals (a chemical compound derived from a natural source, such as food or herbs). The reason for this is for the purpose of possible future regulation in the United States. It would behoove the government to locate these interventions under a single classification, so that a bureau such as the FDA can monitor and regulate the practices. For example, forces such as magnetic fields are studied for effectiveness; the FDA can then monitor and regulate the strength of magnets as required for various effects.

Aromatherapy

Aromatherapy is an intervention that uses essential oils extracted from plants inhaled through the nose to produce relaxation, pain reduction, and alleviation of conditions such as bronchitis. Thirty-one studies were reviewed from Medline, two of which were literature reviews. One of these reviews (Cooke and Ernst, 2000) used statistical analysis in a meta-analysis format. This study reported no findings of statistical significance in support of aromatherapy, except to say that there may be an antianxiety effect of aromatherapy massage. Of the thirty-one studies reviewed, eighteen showed possible positive results in favor of aromatherapy in use or therapeutic application, animal study, or study of the mechanism of action. Seven studies indicated inconclusive results and six showed no findings for support of efficacy.

One of the problems with all of the aromatherapy research was the lack of either a control group or the use of randomization. It is also clear from the review that the British concept of aromatherapy is inclusive of massage, whereas the U.S. concept considers massage a separate component. One study separated aromatherapy versus non-aromatherapy massage (Wilkinson et al., 1999) and found that aromatherapy massage enhanced the therapeutic effect of massage and improved both physical and psychological symptoms. Other problems with aromatherapy research included the lack of differentiation between topical use (both in vitro and as applied to the skin of patients) and inhalation, and the sensitivity that repeated exposure could cause in both patients and practitioners.

One study at the University of Miami School of Medicine (Diego, et al., 1998) found lab indicators (electroencephalogram or EEG results) that demonstrated an effect on mood and performance in math work. Significant effect was shown for lavender to relax and to increase math computation accuracy, and for rosemary to cause faster computation (but not more accurate), with a feeling of less anxiety.

The research did indicate clear trends of usefulness for relaxation and the ability to positively affect mood and behavior in patients, including an increased sense of well-being, decreased stress levels, and improved sleeping patterns. The essential oil most studied was lavender. Much more study needs to be done to determine whether inhalants have antimicrobial and pain-reduction properties.

Herbs

Herbs have been used medicinally for centuries in virtually all cultures. This practice grew simultaneously in places as unrelated as India and North America although neither continent knew the other existed. Although this may not constitute double-blind or any other type of scientific validation, it does constitute an enormous history of vast clinical acceptance and application. We must consider that this has occurred for a reason. The use of herbs is so pancultural and so pervasive in the medical traditions of all the peoples of the world that this significance alone must indicate some very deep and endemic truths about health, health care, and humanity's relationship to these concepts. Dictionaries define neither *herbal medicine* nor *herbology,* but they do define *herbalist.* Philologically speaking, this places people into a special relationship with herbs. We do not seem to have an official study of it, according to the dictionaries, but we have people who "practice healing by the use of herbs." Although this might seem to prove the unscientific basis of herbal medicine, it shows how healing has been thought of throughout history—as something that uses various substances in conjunction with a healer's intent. The American Herbalists Guild is a well-organized group of professionals whose members are often consulted on the use of herbs, and in the writing of books and articles on herbs. The types of herbal medicine are too numerous to list here but can be classified mostly as the traditional practices of the indigenous peoples of various locales, as well as the combined approaches that occur when people move from place to place, and when cultures mix. Numerous examples exist of guides to herbs. David Hoffmann is a British herbalist, and a well-read author in both the United States and Great Britain. His book, *The New Holistic Herbal* (1992), describes the common approach to herbs, in which various types are ascribed properties to support various systems of the body (e.g., digestive, immune, endocrine, reproductive).

Herbalists often classify individual herbs as food, medicinal, aromatic, or poisonous. The Nutrition Labeling and Education Act of 1990 added "herbs, or similar nutritional substances," to the term "dietary supplement," therefore virtually all herbs are considered food by the U.S. government. To an herbalist, food herbs are used in promoting a general healthful lifestyle (garlic, ginger) and medicinal herbs are used from time to time to treat disease. Poisonous herbs can sometimes have limited medicinal application.

Although an herbalist can be consulted directly, they are not necessarily versed in assessment or diagnosis. By tradition, the herbalist is more of an apothecary, who prepares mixtures based on your specifications or at the request of a health practitioner. Even so, holistic health clinics with herbalists are not common in the United States, probably due to the ability of practitioners to recommend types of herbs or due to the fact that already-prepared mixtures are readily obtainable. For the most part, herbal medicine is either self-prescribed and herbs and supplements are purchased in stores, or recommendations are made by practitioners, such as naturopaths and practitioners of Chinese and Ayurvedic medicine. Due to the prevalence of their practice, chiropractors may prescribe more herbs in the United States than any other type of practitioner.

Herbs were used in the early stages of pharmacology, with "active components" being isolated from plants, concentrated, and then administered as a cure (such as foxglove creating the drug digitalis). Pharmacology is based on the assumption that the plant itself must somehow be "simplified" to be most effective (improving on Mother Nature) and on the idea that herbs alone are not strong enough to effect a sufficient change. Today, pharmaceutical drugs are often developed by devising chemical substances that have a specific biochemical reactivity and are not derived from the traditional medicinal use of plants (ethnobotany). A study done by the natural products branch of the National Cancer Institute in 1993 found that more than half of the most important drugs used at that time came from natural plant products (Cassileth, 1998). The use of herbs stands apart from pharmacology in its basic assumption that since the plant is alive, the balance of phytochemicals is more conducive to life and to healing than a concentrated single chemical would be. A current theory (with research in the works) purports that the ways multiple phytochemicals work together within a plant are more effective synergistically than a single chemical derivative alone. This theory raises complicated questions about the standardization of herbs and their effects. Current research in double-blind trials puts effectiveness all over the map for single herbs. This is presumably due to potency and quality in herbs being misunderstood and unregulated. Much more debate and research will have to take place before this can be resolved, however. Herbalist guilds often contend that lack of proper potency is due to unregulated growing techniques and improper gathering times, rather than the quantity of a standardized effective ingredient. Regulating herb farming and harvesting would be considerably more difficult and expensive to perform, but it is necessary if herbal medicine is to remain true to its philosophy.

Some recent success in efficacy has been shown for saw palmetto (prostate enlargement), evening primrose oil (breast pain and pre-menstrual syndrome or PMS), chasteberry (PMS), and ginkgo biloba (memory function) (Keegan, 2001). Other herbs that have been used for centuries, perhaps thousands of years, have also been scientifically substantiated; Cassileth lists fifty-three such herbs (1998). Some of these substances have consistently been used at home (licorice, peppermint) or sold in pharmacies (senna, witch hazel) for various medicinal purposes regardless of scientific substantiation. This is probably due to the fact that many of these herbs appeal to our taste, and others have been used and considered effective by thousands of people, thus keeping their sales constant.

However, with clinical application spanning centuries, it is little wonder that so many herbs have been proven effective by recent scientific studies. Many more herbs will undoubtedly join the ranks of those proven effective. No practitioner or patient will want to be left uneducated or puzzled over their possible uses.

Diet/Vitamins and Minerals/Nutraceuticals

It is perhaps heresy to create a single heading for these things, but in the order listed one flowed from the next, to the next, from a variety of foods we have seemingly always eaten. As with herbal medicine becoming pharmacology, scientists have found out what the actively beneficial components of food are. Of all the things considered complementary and alternative, this area is most closely related to the history of Western science and medicine. The study of biochemistry and the discovery of the Krebs cycle (the metabolic system whereby our bodies derive energy, or "life," from the things we consume) are what led to the study of this area of health. Health food stores and the entire CAM movement can credit much of its impetus to this science. Nutrition has had scant attention by the medical establishment. It had been relegated to nutritionists and nurses—besides, feeding people is nurturing, something that the masculine approach to conventional medicine was happy to leave to the female participants of health care.

The United States Recommended Daily Allowance (USRDA) was introduced by the National Research Council as a means of ensuring that soldiers in World War II were given rations that would prevent severe nutritional deficiencies. As it were, this firmly established the idea for the need for vitamins and other nutrients in our culture. This government body played the role for nutrients that placebo-controlled studies did for pharmaceuticals. It should be recalled that government regulations were instituted to prove safety and effectiveness, but the political demand to establish regulation was based on safety issues, and the ability that some drugs have to maim (thalidomide) and kill (elixir of sulfanilamide). These laws were enacted in 1938, and extended in 1962 (mostly because of the two parenthetical drugs in the previous sentence). Nutrients, on the other hand, presumably do not have the same safety issues, and have never required such a level of scientific study. In 1994, the U.S. Congress passed the Dietary Supplement Health and Education Act, which regulated the dietary supplement industry but also firmly defined supplements as food, removing them from the possibility of being regulated as drugs, and thus, nutraceuticals became the name of pharmaceutically derived nutrients for sale (USFDA, 1999). In theory, if *any* substance could be found in food and isolated, it could become a nutraceutical available over the counter in the United States. In Japan, for instance, the supplement Coenzyme Q10 (CoQ10) is regulated as a drug.

As mentioned, research in nutrition has a long and well-established history. The AMA regularly recognizes the role and efficacy of various nutrients in health. Studies showing the role of cholesterol in heart disease are landmark. Little mention needs to be made of studies to convince either health care professionals or the public about the importance of nutrition. *How* nutrition is important, the proper use of dietary supplements, and such ideas as megavitamin therapy, however, are other matters.

Ayurveda, for example, places digestion above nutrition in importance. In other words, the efficiency of human digestion is responsible for deriving enough life force from the food for survival, growth, and health. Although this may be true, it does not preclude the idea that deficiencies can exist. Ayurveda relies on an herbal mixture called trikatu which consists of three pungent tastes that aid in digestion. Studies have confirmed that it increases the bioavailability of drugs and possibly nutrients (Atal, Zutshi, and Rao, 1981).

One thing that achieves consensus among medical doctors, nutritionists, and naturopaths is that deficiency in nutrients is harmful and should be remedied. This can be achieved by supplementation. Andrew Weil has advocated the use of large doses of vitamin C before surgery in order to facilitate faster recovery (1996). Barrie Cassileth claims that no proof exists that megavitamin therapy can have any benefit and points to the NIH statement that such therapies for psychological disorders is "unsubstantiated . . . ineffective, harmful and deplorable" (1998, p. 67). Many books do not report on the use of high doses of vitamins, but many recommendations among practitioners exceed the USRDA of these nutrients. It is common for a naturopathic physician to recommend larger-than-USRDA dosages to correct deficiencies, and the availability of larger-than-USRDA doses of nutrients is obvious when one enters any store that sells supplements. Sometimes quantities recommended in the *Nutrition Almanac* (Kirschmann and Kirschmann, 1996) are higher than USRDA recommendations and represent therapeutic test dosages. Readers are advised by the authors to consult a physician familiar with nutritional therapy. Otherwise, the recommendations are all made at USRDA levels.

What, then, is nutritional therapy, and can it include large doses of nutrients in order to produce a positive therapeutic effect? Andrew Weil (1997b) says, "In addition to their basic roles in metabolism, some vitamins, taken in larger amounts, have specific preventive and therapeutic effects that are still ignored by many nutritionists and doctors." When his recommendations are reviewed, however, it is clear that all the fat-soluble recommendations are within the USRDA guidelines. He has even reduced his vitamin C recommendation (Weil, 2001).

In the end, conflicting sources often agree that where proper diet is not adhered to, nutrient supplementation can be beneficial. In the treatment of disease, the latest studies show that such nutrients as vitamin C and zinc can reduce the duration and severity of a cold. Further studies are likely to show that nutrients are effective in the treatment of many other diseases. Whether larger-than-USRDA doses are beneficial is a question that will remain controversial. Erring on the side of caution when trying larger doses is recommended.

Special diets abound in popular culture and also within more arcane complementary and alternative modalities. Each comes with a basic idea or philosophy. There are "low" diets, such as low fat, low sodium, and low carbohydrate. These beg to be summarized with the old adage of moderation. In fact, *every* diet begs to be summarized this way. In several longitudinal studies on longevity, varied diets were evident in centenarians. What was common to all was clearly the small amount of food each ate (Chopra, 1993). Biochemistry does support the idea that the body can derive its energy from a variety of sources, and that it ends up boiling down nutrients to drive the Krebs cycle from a vast variety of molecules (Goldberg, 1999).

Dietary recommendations and the latest USRDA food pyramid recommend that a diet be mostly vegetarian with grains, fruits, and vegetables. Vegetarians are adamant that purely vegetarian diets are more healthful. This recommendation is made by systems as old as Ayurveda, where meat is considered "tamasic" (dark/tainted). These beliefs are likely to come from the fact that meat and dairy can and do house more illness-causing microorganisms than other foods. From a zoological and archaeological standpoint, humans are quite capable of consuming and digesting meat, and the species has evolved doing so. However, the Ornish et al. Lifestyle Heart Trial that took place over five years showed marked improvement in indicators such as percent diameter coronary artery stenosis in the research group, and LDL cholesterol levels for persons on a vegetarian diet. This was despite the fact that the control group took lipid-lowering drugs (Keegan, 2001). The research group also made sure their fat intake was no higher than 10 percent, managed stress, attended support groups, and engaged in aerobic exercise. It is unknown how this combination created the improved results, and how strong a role the vegetarian diet played. Moderation appears to be an important consideration in the consumption of meat in human health; however, moral, environmental, and political considerations apply to diet as well. Legitimate environmental concerns include disappearing forests, the amount of land and fossil fuels required to raise meat- and dairy-producing animals, and the morality of killing to eat when it is not technically necessary for many peoples to do so.

The different kinds of diets cannot all be dealt with in this work, but the macrobiotic diet is worth mentioning because of its popularity and potential usefulness. Originally, the diet consisted entirely of brown rice. This was found to be insufficient and a cause of malnutrition. Later, the diet was modified to a largely vegetarian diet of predominantly whole grains and beans with occasional fish allowed. The benefits of this diet are not out of line with the previously mentioned food pyramid of the USRDA recommendations. This modified macrobiotic diet is most effective for mid- to later-life persons who need to lower fat and cholesterol intake. It is not recommended for young adults approaching child-rearing age, pregnant women, or children. Studies in the United States, Belgium, Norway, and the Netherlands have corroborated serious deficiencies from the diet, including nutritional rickets with breathing abnormalities, bone deformities, vitamin B_{12} deficiency, growth retardation, deficiencies of proteins, vitamins, calcium, and riboflavin, leading to retarded growth and slower psychomotor development (Cassileth, 1998). It is not clear whether these studies were for the brown rice-only diet, or included the stricter ratios of 50 to 60 percent grains, 5 percent miso-based soups, 25 to 30 percent vegetables, and 5 to 10 percent beans and sea vegetables. It is highly unlikely that a macrobiotic diet that includes fish and occasional supplementation from other food groups would create such severe problems.

Magnetic/Electrical/Electromagnetic Interventions

According to the NIH, these interventions are included in an "energy" domain with such modalities as shamanism. However, since the claims for the energy of a magnet, or magnetic strength, are not at all similar to the metaphysical claims of a shaman's ability to intervene in the spirit world, it is included here as part of the biologically based domain. Magnetic, electrical, and electromagnetic energies can be measured in Western scientific terms. These energies can be dosed and administered to attempt a specific physical intervention. The main reason for this classification here is that all biologically based interventions would come under the jurisdiction of the FDA. If any agency should regulate, classify strength, and make dosage recommendations, this is the agency. Although these interventions are neither foods nor drugs per se, the effect desired is biologically based.

Magnetic therapy has been adopted from Asian practices where the Japanese have used them for a considerable length of time. After an explosion of interest in magnetic therapy in the United States in the early to mid-1990s, a reputable study was conducted in 1997 at Baylor College of Medicine, Houston, Texas. Researchers tested magnet therapy on patients with painful postpolio syndrome. Real and placebo magnets (credit-card sized sheets with no magnetic properties) were used. Seventy-six percent of the patients receiving the magnets said they had less pain. Only 19 percent of those who received the placebos had the same results (Almond, 1997).

Carlos Vallbona, MD, conducted the study. He did not discover the mechanism whereby this occurred, but suggests that electromagnetic fields may somehow alter the processing of pain signals. Other theories include the possibility (1) that magnets work by interacting with the iron in blood cells and by improving the blood's oxygen-carrying ability; (2) that they stimulate nerve endings; or (3) that they modify other electrical processes in the body.

JAMA reported the ineffectiveness of magnets in March of 2000 (Collacott et al., 2000), but medical doctors disagree on both their effectiveness and their possible use. By August of 2000, *JAMA* published a well-referenced letter from Craig Burkhart, MSPH, MD (Medical College of Ohio, Toledo). Dr. Burkhart cites theories of effectiveness based on clear laboratory observations. No fewer than four physicians responded with well-researched disputes to the negative study in the August 2000 issue's letters to the editor section (Burkhart et al., 2000). Clearly, a dispute over the possibility of magnets' effectiveness exists that *JAMA* is willing to air. This is an example of an intervention that does not come clearly from the "other side"—the CAM side—of the aisle. It will be interesting to see whether a similar embrace by established medical practice occurs for magnets as has occurred with acupuncture. If so, it will be another addition of an Asian-based modality.

Electrical and electromagnetic forces are applied for similar reasons as magnets. The electrical and electromagnetic stimulation of muscle tissue and its subsequent release to cause muscle relaxation and to reduce spasm is well applied in medical, osteopathic, and chiropractic offices. These methods have been found effective, depending on the way in which the charge is delivered (Weil, 1999). Again, it is suggested here that such interventions be classified with dosage recommendations and any required regulations be made by the FDA.

BODY-BASED MANIPULATION THERAPIES

This domain of CAM houses two original U.S. health care therapies, which are now fully licensed and almost fully accepted forms of care: osteopathy and chiropractic. It is also the home for the traditionally accepted therapeutic technique of massage. Despite some specific practices within each of these modalities, this domain is the least disputed and most used complementary domain. Even reflexology (massage of the hands or feet based on the belief that pressure applied to specific points on these extremities benefits other parts of the body as a reflexive response through the nervous system), which lacks significant study, is sometimes recommended as a complementary method due to its low risk and ability to cause deep relaxation. Each of these modalities deserves a closer look, even those with a less stringent review of scientific evidence.

Bodywork/Massage

Massage has a long history in virtually all cultures of the world. Its application is rich and varied, and encompasses a vast array of techniques that are only briefly summarized here. The encompassing term "bodywork" involves therapeutic touch or manipulation of the body by various specialized techniques, including those used in chiropractic and osteopathy. Its application is accepted now by both CAM and conventional medicine as being effective for relieving tension, anxiety, and pain. A 1995 medical journal reported also that patients receiving pediatric massage "got well sooner" (Cassileth, 1998). However, not all types of massage and bodywork listed in Table 1.2 are considered research validated.

As evidenced in Table 1.2, not all CAM modalities are classified clearly and easily within the five domains. Some bodywork incorporates mind/body techniques to achieve results and therefore resists classification.

A search of Medline produced eight studies for foot reflexology. An Austrian study looked at mechanisms of action for foot reflexology (Sudmeier et al., 1999). The study reviewed changes of renal blood flow during organ-associated foot reflexology as measured by color Doppler sonography. Peak velocity of the blood flow to the right and left kidneys was studied when kidney reflex points were stimulated. This placebo-controlled study revealed a marked improvement in the vascular resistance index, decreasing significantly in real versus sham reflexology.

Of the other seven reflexology studies, six found positive statistical change for problems concerning pain, tension, bowel movement, and PMS. Some of this change was statistically significant. The one dissenting study showed an effect for foot reflexology as compared to

TABLE 1.2. Types of Bodywork and Massage

Type of Bodywork	Description
Traditional Massage	Research-validated traditional massage is taught by schools accepted by organizations such as the American Massage Therapy Association.
Chinese/ Ayurvedic	Asian cultures incorporate massage as an important part of their treatment regimens. Both Ayurvedic and Chinese massage rely on application of pressure to various acupressure or "marma" points. Meditation and patient participation via breath work is an important part of these applications.
Reflexology	CAM purists will dispute classifying reflexology as massage. However, it is based on the application of pressure to various reflex points. Although developed separately from Chinese medicine, modern reflexology utilizes the Chinese system of meridians and can therefore be classified as massage. As a diagnostic technique it cannot be classified this way, but most reflexologists no longer attempt to practice diagnosis.
Craniosacral Therapy	This therapy is credited to both chiropractors and osteopaths, and is aimed at the base of the skull and the lower back and buttocks area. The theory is that when spinal fluids surrounding these areas are manipulated, pain and tension are released.
Deep-Tissue Massage	Works to restore deep connective tissue and circulatory function. Also used in multiple sclerosis. Often attributed to the Swedish massage tradition.
Rolfing	Based on yoga, the Alexander technique, and osteopathy. Rolfing was developed by Ida P. Rolf and uses exercise, hand manipulation, and equipment to affect deep changes to the fascia.
Hellerwork	Combines Rolfing-like techniques with emotional counseling, which may underlay physical problems.
Myofascial Release	Similar to Rolfing and Hellerwork, but not set up in multiple sessions. Uses single techniques, which may or may not be repeated.
Movement	Several of these and other therapies incorporate the idea of reeducation in movement to improve pain and flexibility as well as to prevent future problems.
Suggestion and Visualization	Techniques such as Rubenfeld Synergy and some of these techniques use forms of hypnosis, visualization, and psychotherapy to further extend therapeutic intent.

the relaxing effect of simple foot massage, but said that it was detrimental in abdominal postsurgical situations in gynecology. Perhaps this was due to an overstimulation of the bowels from reflexology. All the studies were completed from 1993 to 2000. No study replications were listed.

Massage and bodywork techniques are rich and varied. There appears to be little disagreement that they are ultimately effective for relaxation and pain relief.

Chiropractic

This modality has the least illustrious history because it was founded in the late nineteenth century by D. D. Palmer, an uneducated laborer, and made into a mail-order financial empire by his disreputable son. The founder's grandson began reversing its bad name, established schools, and began the political process for licensing. Chiropractic practitioners in the United States understood early on the need to engage in the politics of health care, and in a mere 100 years, established the practice with licensing in all fifty states. Although osteopathy accomplished this, it did so by basing itself on conventional medical care. Chiropractic did so while being staunchly opposed by the AMA. In 1972, the Medicare Act was amended to include chiropractic (Keegan, 2001). In 1992, a study by the Rand Corporation examined twenty-two clinical trials and concluded that chiropractic is effective for various types of lower back pain (Cassileth, 1998). Finally, in 1994, an independent panel from the Agency for Health Care Policy and Research concluded that "chiropractic is the most effective treatment for acute lower back pain" (Keegan, 2001, p. 242). Although chiropractics' claims are for a much broader range of benefit than lower back pain, this particular study ends the purported idea that chiropractic is not beneficial for any reason.

Thousands of persons have gone to chiropractors, have claimed benefit, and have recommended the procedure to friends and families, making chiropractic the most sought-after alternative in medicine in the United States. Despite the lack of randomized clinical trial, it is unlikely that this exhaustive clinical application over the past 100 years would prove inconclusive in regard to its efficacy.

Chiropractic has now moved into directions in medicine that incorporate post-Newtonian laws of physics (which is good, since these discoveries have been around since 1900). These ideas include the theory that entropy, or deterioration in systems, is caused not only by gravity and the wear of friction over time, but also by the "memory" that the body's systems hold within themselves, of thoughts and emotional impact borne by the larger organism. Memory is given a specific quantum role in health. Chiropractic's founder may have been naive in some respects, but his idea that the spine is the central location of life, both physical and metaphysical, is a belief also found in Ayurveda. The practice of yoga is centered on the spine, and meditations involving the chakras (located where nadis or energy meridians intersect) are considered essential in drawing together mind, body, and spirit. Standard chiropractic does not embrace this particular view, but it is noteworthy that a separate culture arrived at similar conclusions to the spine's role in health thousands of years before. Recent developments in chiropractic practice combine these ideas in physics with beliefs about the spine to create a theory called "network chiropractic." It contends that trapped negativity (physical injuries, emotions) becomes ensconced in the human nervous system and can be released through manipulation of the spine. Network chiropractic is a term coined by Dr. Donald Epstein, a New York City chiropractor, and is not a new theory but rather the coming together of holistic ideas that many chiropractors have used for years. These ideas incorporate lifestyle and spiritual ideas with an emphasis on emotional healing.

Osteopathy

Osteopathy is considered complementary or alternative today only in its manipulation of the soft tissue and bones. Most osteopaths do not practice this manipulation; they instead practice medicine in a way that is identical to medical doctors.

Osteopathy was also discovered or created by a single physician in 1874, Andrew Taylor Still. Osteopathy does differ slightly from Western medicine in philosophy and approach, as it considers the body a collection of systems that work together. Osteopaths must receive additional training beyond the standard and required MD in order to become licensed in osteopathy in all fifty states. Osteopaths are the only other type of medical practitioners in the United States, besides medical doctors, who may prescribe controlled medications.

Osteopathic manipulation hovers in the same range as chiropractic and massage for effectiveness in pain relief.

ENERGY/METAPHYSICAL THERAPIES

As mentioned in the biologically based section, this classification strays from the NIH model by excluding the clearly measurable electromagnetic energies and including only the currently immeasurable and metaphysical ones. This classification has been, on the surface, the most confusing and controversial in CAM because it includes such areas as faith healing and shamanism. However, the arguments against such interventions as quackery and charlatanry have been effectively brought down.

Therapeutic Touch/Reiki

For the purposes of this book, Reiki and therapeutic touch are classified together as interventions that claim to use or direct metaphysical energy in order to aid in relaxation and heal disease. In both practices, practitioners hold their hands above or place their hands lightly on the recipient in order to direct this energy.

In 1998, *JAMA* published an article on the results of a study on therapeutic touch that was conducted in 1996 and 1997 by an unusual investigator: a nine-year-old student. The article was written by Linda Rosa, BSN, RN, from the Questionable Nurse Practices Task Force, National Council Against Health Fraud, Inc., Loma Linda, California. It has unusual co-authors for scientific investigations as well, one of whom is concerned exclusively with quackery (Stephen Barrett, a retired Allentown, Pennsylvania psychiatrist) (Rosa et al., 1998). As in a study previously discussed in the section on homeopathy, it involved the magician James Randi. It is probably safe to say that Ms. Rosa, Dr. Barrett, and Mr. Randi were not looking for evidence to confirm efficacy but rather to extend their work on quackery and fraud. To add even more interest to the story, the nine-year-old who conducted the study was Emily Rosa, the daughter of Linda Rosa. Although Linda Rosa claims she had nothing to do with encouraging her daughter to work on such a project, it is clear that the daughter was imitating the defrauding work of her mother. The study concluded that "no well-designed study demonstrates any health benefit from therapeutic touch," which is in stark contrast to the findings of Dolores Krieger, Professor Emeritus of Nursing Science at New York University. Krieger criticized the study as "poor in terms of design and methodology," citing that the study's designer should not have conducted it, and that the twenty-one subjects used were an insufficient and unrepresentative number. She also noted that "innumerable clinical studies" show therapeutic touch to be effective—some of which are later quoted in this section (Hinman and Richards, 1998). A huge number of letters were also written to *JAMA* in protest of the study and its methodology. The last reference to the 1998 article was in 1999 at which point it was still being defended by its authors in follow-up statements published in *JAMA*. We can assume the AMA published these follow-ups to be certain it got the last word in on how it stands as a professional organization toward therapeutic touch (TT).

The mainstream press picked up on this story and screamed headlines suggesting that a little girl "debunked" TT, playing both on the youth of the investigator and the fact that she was female. It was clear that the message passed here was: even a young child is smart enough to figure out that TT is bogus—so bogus that even a little girl can prove it. To be sure, the original article does not appear to contain the sex bias (it does contain the age bias), but the subsequent press treatment played on the student's sex as well.

This is one of the best examples of the "camps" for and against CAM in recent documentation. Although the desired effect was to debunk this longtime practice of nurses, it raised the emotional ire of scores of intelligent physicians, nurses, and investigators (both female and male) who wrote to *JAMA* to say that they were, indeed, not as smart as this *little girl*.

As will be discussed in the following section on prayer, it will seem unreasonable to accept the clearly positive research results on the intentions of prayer, and say that they do not apply to the intentions in any of the metaphysical modalities, including TT. Clearly, something more significant is occurring here in regard to health care than the opportunity that was taken by defrauders and debunkers to try to lay waste to an ancient nursing tradition. Practitioners of TT make it clear that healing intent occurs in TT, similar to prayer.

Since TT has been a longtime tradition of nurses, it is difficult to find criticism of the practice in works by nurses, even in the rather conservative work of Barrie Cassileth. Dr. Cassileth (1998) states, "No objective, scientific studies about Therapeutic Touch have been published in reputable journals." Is she suggesting that journals such as *Nursing Research* (Keller and Bzdek, 1986) and *Nursing Science Quarterly* (Meehan, 1993) are not reputable journals? This seems doubtful.

A Medline Internet search conducted on May 31, 2001, yielded 335 records for TT. Of these, thirty-one reported on clinical studies of the efficacy of TT or lab indicators for physiological change in subjects receiving TT. Of the twenty-seven clinical studies, nineteen showed TT to be effective in some way, three showed TT to be "not effective," and five showed inconclusive results. Of these studies, one meta-analysis (Winstead-Fry and Kijek, 1999) and two literature reviews (Spence and Olson, 1997; Easter, 1997) all reported efficacy for TT. If these are from "disreputable" journals one has to question why they are listed on Medline, which is used for research information by health professionals worldwide. The fact is that plenty of research and evidence exists, despite consistency and quality questions (questions which arise in all scientific inquiry), to suggest that TT is both useful and effective. The greatest amount of evidence supports its ability to cause relaxation. Both quantitative studies (Sneed et al., 2001; Wordell and Engebretson, 2001) have shown lab indicator evidence for physiological change pointing toward relaxation and improved immune function, and pretest and posttest data for subjects clearly show greater relaxation, improved mood, and improved quality of life.

Prayer, Shamanism, and Spirit in Medicine

Research into the effects of prayer over the past twenty years has changed the way science validates metaphysical effects, even if it has not changed the attitudes of patients and practitioners alike.

Larry Dossey's 1999 book *Reinventing Medicine* summarizes these studies. The idea of individual or group prayer for the sick is familiar to anyone who has attended church in the last 2,000 years. In fact, when the AMA was actively creating medical licensing laws in the 1860s, the clergy was exempted from being disallowed to diagnose or treat disease (Weil, 1995). In his book, Dossey describes a "fantasy emergency room" that uses prayer groups from around the world and from all religions—Christian, Jewish, Hindu—to make what he terms "nonlocal" intercession. This uses multiple religions to request intercession from an outside metaphysical power. Dossey is unique when he talks about the physician in charge "inviting" the same type of nonlocal mind (the term Dossey coined for how mind and intent influenced the physical) to aid and speed the healing of the patient. Dossey recommends that physicians intercede on behalf of their patients with the realm of nonlocal mind in the same way shamans intercede in the spiritual realm on behalf of their patients.

Dossey presents his work in the context of commonly accepted Western scientific techniques for determining efficacy. He makes several extremely important points, which are summarized here.

1. The author discloses 150 studies of prayer.
2. Meta-analysis of the studies shows small but clinical significance in improvement for the prayed-for group in study after study.
3. Small clinical significance should not be taken lightly. Many medications are approved with little therapeutic effect: The effects of prayer are proven to a greater extent in clinical studies than the meta-analysis of aspirin's effect in preventing heart disease.
4. Dossey expresses the odds of things happening randomly versus through the effect of nonlocal mind. For example, when he discussed an experiment in which healers "intended" the growth of yeast cells to increase, he states the chances were less than two in 10,000 that such a result could have occurred by chance.

Dossey delivers some excellent historical work uncovering how some of the greatest scientific minds worked, and how they used thinking techniques that could be considered nonlocal. He describes the intuitive techniques of Jonas Salk, inventor of the polio vaccine, who, when pondering the immune system, would mentally crawl into an immune system and imagine what it was like on a cellular level to combat virus or cancer foes.

It is insightful and somewhat poignant when Dossey tells us that only about 15 percent of medical diagnoses are based on lab tests. "The rest of the time, we physicians rely on subjective reasons—including hunches and premonitions—in making diagnoses, deciding which tests should be ordered and selecting treatments" (Dossey, 1999, p. 20). Although many physicians and scientists purport that health techniques today are backed up with scientific proof, it seems that arriving at health conclusions of diagnoses still relies on an artistic blend of lab tests, knowledge, experience, and intuition. Does prudence require the use of all the techniques available?

This prudence is described in a marvelous story Dossey tells about Mohandas Gandhi, who had previously refused Western medical intervention in his life as "not natural." An attack of acute appendicitis had Gandhi reconsidering his views, and under the advice of British Surgeon General Colonel Maddock, he consented to surgery. At that point in his life, Gandhi made a decision that allowed for greater inclusiveness of approaches to health. Without it, his death was probably quite certain. Colonel Maddock's confidence must have inspired Gandhi and contributed to the success of the surgery. Gandhi even had documents drawn up to indicate to his followers that the procedure was fully consensual—and he went on to lead one of the most significant political liberations in history.

This play between the physical world and a world of consciousness is where Ayurveda, the traditional health care practice in India, has not been separated from its roots. Ayurveda has a set of very specific explanations for such phenomena, and it is very specific about the play of how this physical world in which we live figures into the equation. According to Ayurveda, consciousness precedes the creation of the physical universe and is the common origin toward which all things are drawn. This explanation gives us the field in which nonlocal mind occurs. In emphasizing the need for physical interventions, Dossey is also noting the Ayurvedic belief that once the physical world was created, it could not be ignored. A force called ahankara came into being, and this is the force that "holds things apart from one another" (it can also be thought of as a physics "ego" in matter identity). Due to this reality, and due to the creation of the universe in which we live, time has also been set into motion and this linear time creates a world of cause and effect. This is why physical elements (or "things," as Dossey calls them) are contained in disease, and why other physical things within this realm will affect and alter disease for a cure as well. Although we may wish to explore the concept of nonlocal mind and meditate on the idea that mind and brain are different things, we must also realize that we have a brain that currently houses this consciousness in its entirety. If not, then the living eyes that are gazing at the words upon this page are not alive at all. When this consciousness leaves the brain, we are simply dead. If Dossey's ideas can be refined, it is the physical manifestations of disease that must be treated with physical interventions, but the state of nonlocal interruption, which brought about the disease in the first place, must be treated through nonlocal means. Similarly, mind/body techniques are most effective when illness is "on the way" and has not yet physically manifested itself. Once it has, we must try to influence the healing of such disease on all levels, as well as strive to prevent its return.

In Ayurveda, the concept of perusha (which can also be thought of as "love seeking to explain itself") is the golden thread that re-attaches itself to the primordial consciousness. It is the condition by which nonlocal mind can function in this world. Ayurveda and yoga offer specific technical systems for bringing this about as well, such as the meditative practices of kundalini and tantra. Explanations of these practices are beyond the scope of this work; however, kundalini techniques are used to "transcend" physical pain, discomfort, and suffering.

CONCLUSION

This chapter has discussed specific modalities in the light of five basic domains of classification for CAM. This framework is not meant to be a perfect or restrictive system for CAM practices, but rather a tool for understanding it and a reference for its possible applications. In review, the five domains can be thought to have a generally effective application summarized in Table 1.3. This chapter has also made reference to the traditional scientific evidence for the efficacy of many of these modalities, while recommending caution in the approach to this scientific evidence, and noting that Western medicine utilizes many techniques that are supported as well, or not even as well, as these CAM modalities.

TABLE 1.3. Practical Applications of the Five Complementary and Alternative Medicine Domains

Domain	Applications
Alternative Medical Systems	These systems provide the roots to many of the other four domains. These are appropriate for persons who are from the cultures in which they originate, and can be applied as complementary and alternative means for treating illnesses not responding to conventional therapies.
Mind/Body Interventions	Recommended to draw the patient into the activity of being responsible for, and being influential in affecting, his or her health.
Biologically Based Interventions	These are extensions of the same type of interventions (especially medication) that conventional medicine uses but are not as readily promoted. The same type of placebo-controlled study as required for medication and surgery can be applied.
Body-Based Manipulation Therapies	These should be used to relax and relieve pain, and as such should be considered as adjunct to all health care. They are also useful to help repair physical damage and to reeducate patients on the use of their bodies.
Energy/Metaphysical Therapies	This element rounds out the entirety of our being and speaks for the "spiritual element" that *JAMA* reported as being one of the main reasons that patients access CAM. It must be explored at the personal comfort level of each individual patient and practitioner, but it must be explored for complete health.

Chapter 2

Research

It is good to know the classifications and latest research results for the efficacy of modalities, but what does the public think? What do physicians think who serve these patients, and what do other health professionals think, especially those who already run health practices, clinics, and programs that incorporate modalities from the five domains? Through original research results, this chapter attempts to answer some of those questions in ways that will stimulate thought for each group.

One of the colossal problems in creating a coordinated practice of CAM is to understand the patients, the thinking of their primary care physicians, and the interests and thinking of the CAM practitioners. To this end, three separate surveys were conducted by the author in 1999: one was made with 438 patients, one with thirty-five physicians who attended them, and one was made with fifty-nine CAM programs. Reports on specific results appear in Appendix A (Patient Raw Data), Appendix B (Physician Raw Data), and Appendix C (Clinic Raw Data).

WHAT HEALTH CARE CONSUMERS THINK

Both the patient and the physician surveys were conducted in conjunction with the Northwest New Jersey Community Action Program (NORWESCAP), Coventry Family Practice of Phillipsburg, New Jersey, and Warren Hospital (the hospital serving the area covered by the survey). NORWESCAP surveyed clients engaged in their Women, Infants, and Children Supplemental Food program (WIC), and both the family practice and hospital surveyed patients and physicians. All three organizations surveyed clients waiting for appointments with physicians and nutritionists during a two-week period in the spring of

1999. Although coordinating the survey with three organizations produced significant numbers of responses, it accordingly limited the randomness of the sample to clients of these programs. Comparisons to larger national surveys reported in *JAMA,* however, demonstrate that the results are similar enough to suggest that the sample was representative. The questions were developed by a committee of five persons including—in addition to representatives of NORWESCAP, Coventry Family Practice, and Warren Hospital—a retired member of the Methodist clergy, and the president of the Center for Natural Healing, a CAM program in Washington, New Jersey. This method proved to be highly effective in covering the concerns, interests, and needs of a diverse group.

For the purposes of this book, patients or health care consumers are considered the most important group interested in CAM. The CAM paradigm in health has been called a consumer revolution and this flies in the face of the traditional model of being a patient. The root of the word *patient* implies someone who remains patient while physicians and health care practitioners "do something to them" in order to improve their health. This "doing" and the lack of patient patience have caused not only the consumer revolution of CAM but also the increasingly litigious nature of patients. Both the attitudes of physicians who "do" and the patients who allow things to be done need a serious adjustment as we enter the twenty-first century. Chapter 5 discusses the patient/physician relationship and ideas for decreasing litigation as suggested by this research.

When chiropractic and the purchase of vitamins are included, the number of persons that *JAMA* says consume CAM constitutes 30 to 50 percent of the population in industrialized nations (Astin et al., 1998). The patient survey conducted here found that 287 persons of 438 (66 percent) used nutritional supplements or herbs, or engaged in some CAM modality. The demographics that this survey covered can be seen in Appendix A. Absolutely no correlation was shown between interest in alternative and complementary therapies, and either education or income levels *at all.* This suggests that CAM use is equally regarded due to a cultural acceptance that is beyond what has been previously considered. The only slight difference in the demographics tracked appears to be for the age group of thirty to fifty. This group is 6 percent more interested in the complementary therapies than the average of the entire sample. Since they are a large part of the aging population, and health difficulties increase as a rule with age, paying attention to this growing trend in alternative and complementary health might be wise. Just over 50 percent reported taking nutritional supplements.

An insignificantly larger amount (52 percent) reported taking prescriptions or over-the-counter (OTC) medication. This indicates a trend toward both of these "pill-form" health interventions. One hundred twenty-nine (57 percent) of the 225 people taking vitamins also take one or more prescribed or OTC drugs, so the chance is higher that patients will take medication if they also take vitamins. Are people replacing drugs with herbs? Twelve percent of patients surveyed reported taking herbs, and of those forty people, 27 (or 67.5 percent) were also taking medication at the same time. These statistics seem to indicate that the public feels that these therapies are complementary rather than alternative. Perhaps there need not be "camps" of CAM versus Western medicine in health care. Competition between CAM and the medications used in conventional medicine may not be necessary: cross marketing might be recommended.

Conditions with which patients suffered were various, with 32 percent reporting being overweight. A clear correlation was shown between poor nutrition and being overweight and, not surprisingly, patients wished to learn about nutrition more than about any other CAM modality. Anxiety and headaches respectively rounded out the top three complaints of the patient respondents. It is this question of anxiety, if successfully addressed, that can alleviate the reduction in quality of life.

The group of patients surveyed used specific types of nutritional supplements and herbs. Significant numbers of people consumed multivitamins, vitamins B, C, and E, and calcium (see Appendix A). Folic acid was also separately reported, presumably because of the large number of prenatal women who were part of the study. Although the number of people taking herbal supplements was also significant (forty people or 11.67 percent), the numbers reported for individual herbs were not sufficient to outline any trends. However, St. John's wort topped the list, with five people reporting its consumption. Herbs reported as being consumed by more than one person included echinacea, black cohosh, ginseng, chamomile, feverfew, garlic, ginkgo biloba, and juniper berry. Physicians reported prescribing St. John's wort more than any other herb, demonstrating the power of media to create a demand for supplements. This survey was taken in 1999, and press coverage just before this time touted St. John's wort as an effective antidepressant. This illustrates some of the confusion suffered by patients and physicians alike about CAM. Herbalists from the American Herbalists Guild would recommend the use of St. John's wort in conjunction with lemon balm for depression. In herbalist practice, it is not considered effective without this herbal partner. Yet St. John's wort was consumed without lemon balm by these people.

Interesting correlations exist between reported illnesses and whether or not a patient consumes nutritional or herbal supplements. Table 2.1 illustrates that those interested in CAM are more likely to be suffering from particular health problems. There is little or no significant correlation between the consumption of nutritional supplements and reported illness when the supplement-consumer's sample is compared to the general sample. However, significant differences occur for those who consume herbal supplements: consumers of herbs are more likely to report trouble with anxiety, fatigue, arthritis, interpersonal relationships, and the heart. No correlation was found with the type of herb consumed and these conditions. Moreover, it may be concluded that persons suffering from these conditions are generally looking for health answers outside the realm of conventional health and are therefore willing to use these interventions in their quest for relief.

No significant differences in reported illnesses were found with those not consuming supplements when compared with the general sample, but significant differences were found when consumers of either herbs and nutritional supplements were compared to those who did not consume any supplements. A trend was evident when consumption of supplements and drugs was compared to nonconsumption. Table 2.1 shows this as a succession from wellness to illness from left to right, with those taking nothing reporting less illness.

A large statistical difference occurs between the rate of reported illness for those who consume nothing at all and those who take medications. There might be nothing to this, except that the progression toward reported illness is so distinct for so many individual illnesses that influencing factors must exist. In Germany, it is required by law to start with milder interventions and progress to strong medications in treatment. What may be evident by this progression is that patients in the United States are also inclined to take a course from no treat-

TABLE 2.1. Strategies to Deal with Illnesses (Percent) (n = 437)

Illness	Take Nothing	Do not Take Meds	Use Neither Herbs nor Vitamins	Use Vitamins	Use Herbs	Take Meds
Overweight	19.00	22.63	30.99	32.73	35.00	42.73
Headaches	16.00	15.26	21.60	19.55	20.00	25.99
Allergy	12.00	15.26	16.90	19.09	15.00	20.70
Anxiety	11.00	13.68	20.66	21.36	37.50	29.07
Asthma	11.00	8.42	13.15	8.64	12.50	14.10
Fatigue	7.00	8.42	11.74	14.09	22.50	17.62
Interpersonal Relations	5.00	5.26	5.63	8.64	17.50	9.69
Sinusitis	3.00	4.21	8.45	10.45	12.50	14.98
Irritable Bowel	2.00	3.68	3.29	6.36	7.50	6.17
Attention Deficit	2.00	2.11	1.88	2.27	0.00	2.20
High Blood Pressure	1.00	2.11	16.90	16.36	15.00	29.52
Arthritis	0.00	4.74	7.04	13.64	15.00	15.42
High Cholesterol	0.00	1.58	5.63	11.36	7.50	14.54
Heart	0.00	1.58	6.10	9.55	12.50	13.66
Diabetes	0.00	0.53	4.69	8.18	7.50	11.45
Osteoporosis	0.00	0.00	0.94	3.18	0.00	3.96
Cancer	0.00	0.00	0.94	0.91	0.00	1.76
Fibromyalgia	0.00	0.00	0.47	0.45	2.50	0.88
Average % of reported illnesses	**4.94**	**6.08**	**9.83**	**11.49**	**13.33**	**15.25**

ment, through nutritional supplements and herbs, to medication as their wellness level deteriorates. This table might also suggest that certain conditions, such as overweight, fatigue, and high blood pressure, are factors in other illnesses and require that persons suffering from these conditions receive more treatment for these and other illnesses. Another possible factor in why these reported illnesses increase as interventions also increase is that the interventions themselves may be causative of those and related illnesses! This survey lacks sufficient information to answer these questions, but it is logical to infer that as people feel more ill, they seek stronger and stronger treatments.

The preferred place to purchase supplements by patients was reported as the pharmacy, followed closely by the grocery store. Physicians directed their patients to purchase supplements at the pharmacy but recommended health food stores over grocery stores. This probably indicates that pharmacies are thought of as being the best location to purchase pill-form interventions, and that grocery stores are convenient places to pick up supplements (being thought of as something that is consumed often, as is food).

The types of CAM used by patients fell within a broad range, with at least one person reporting that he or she used each listed modality (see Appendix A), except for naturopathy. The largest group (23 percent) claimed prayer as a complementary choice. This intervention does not require the participation of anyone other than the patient, and prayer is taught as part of Western religious traditions. Many church congregations incorporate community prayer time on Sundays with congregation members filling out prayer cards, often expressing concerns over the health of other church members. Although this intervention is somewhat passive, pastoral counseling ranked sixth on the list of nineteen interventions, truly making metaphysical considerations the *highest* for patients when considering complementary and alternative methods. CAM group practices currently offer metaphysical interventions the least, presumably because they are offered through the patient's religious affiliations, but CAM practitioners should consider this type of metaphysical intervention an important part of any health plan.

Another intervention chosen by many respondents is music/art therapy (9 percent). It is not believed that patients in this survey formally engaged in music or art therapy with a trained professional, but that they expressed the use of music and art to alleviate conditions and promote their well-being. This should be viewed by CAM practitioners as an opportunity to utilize and focus this desire through the incorporation of professionally guided music and art therapy as part of an overall health plan. Western culture has used drama and art since the time of the ancient Greek Asclepions (healing temples), and this may indicate that the practice has never died out within our culture (Keegan, 2001).

Where patients learned about CAM was interesting. Most reported learning from the media (newspapers/radio/TV), then from family physicians, the Internet, magazines, and practitioners of various forms of CAM. This trend shows a continued respect for the family physician but also indicates the increasing independence of patients. The use of the media for health information may indicate a lack of time or a lack of desire to spend time researching on their own. This indicates the need for media to be particularly careful in its reporting habits, and opens the door for CAM practitioners to establish relationships with the media, even if it is to urge the public to become educated about health through means in addition to the media. This may not be as much of a problem as it seems, because most people reported wanting to learn about CAM from CAM practitioners first, and then from their family physicians. Still, the media placed high as a selected mode of health education, and taking the time to research and attend seminars may be more of an idealistic urge of the public.

Half as many people reported using the Internet to find CAM information as those who reported using newspaper, radio, and television, which still constitutes 25 percent of the sample. The Internet has quickly become accepted as an information source, and it is probably assumed to be accurate by most of its users. However, the Internet, when used to search the World Wide Web with various search engines, can lead health care consumers to sites that appear authoritative but are not. Just as likely, the search engines may direct individuals to the advertisers that pay the most money to have their sites listed first in the search results. This is fine if consumers understand they are reading someone's opinion. However, the amount of misinformation is dangerous, such as the tendency for the World Wide Web to perpetuate urban legends—fascinating or interesting-sounding stories or "facts" that make dire predictions and issue stern warnings but have no basis in reality. On the other hand, the Internet is replete with authoritative resources of correct facts and informed opinions that can aid the health care consumer in weighing ideas and evidence when making their own health-related decisions. The sheer volume of information now available to the general public with a few clicks of the mouse is unprecedented, and is undoubtedly a large contributor to the health care consumer's independence.

The top interests of patients should be placed on the educational outreach plan of all CAM practices. These include nutrition, massage, mind/body interventions, music/art, yoga, meditation, herbs, and aromatherapy. It is most important to note that significant interest was expressed in seventeen of the nineteen areas listed. The last two areas of expressed interest were for Ayurveda and naturopathy. Since these were also reported as little used, this does not mean that the public is uninterested but probably that they require additional information to become interested and eventually to accept these modalities.

Seventy-four people, or 47 percent of those interested in learning about CAM, did not report using any sort of CAM, meaning that a large percentage of people are ready and willing to learn before starting the use of any modality. When coupled with their selected number-one way of learning—through a seminar by a practitioner of a modality—it strongly suggests that all CAM practitioners make public seminars a part of their practice.

Table 2.2 compares the patients' CAM interests and activities engaged in, the physicians' CAM interests and referrals, and the modalities offered by CAM practices. Programs and practices that offer CAM should take into account the patients' interests in consuming CAM modalities. Still, they should keep a watchful eye on the interests of physicians as well.

The surveys all suggest that neither physicians nor CAM programs have a clear understanding of what the public desires, nor why certain modalities are desired.

PHYSICIANS

The Stanford Center for Research in Disease Prevention reviewed twenty-five surveys conducted between 1982 and 1995 that studied how physicians felt about, referred to, and actually used the CAM therapies of acupuncture, chiropractic, homeopathy, herbal medicine, and massage. Six studies were not used because the authors did not feel the methodologies of the studies were valid (Astin et al., 1998).

All the surveys reported acupuncture as the highest rate of referral for physicians (43 percent). Chiropractic was referred to by 40 percent and massage had 21 percent of physicians referring to it as a therapy. The actual rate that physicians themselves practiced CAMs in the report was 9 percent for homeopathy and 19 percent for chiropractic and massage therapy combined. About half of the physicians

TABLE 2.2. The Interests in CAM of Patients Ranked from Greatest to Least, and Compared to the Interests of Physicians and the Offering of CAM Programs (Percent)

Modality	Practice and Interests of Patients	Referrals and Interests of Physicians	What CAM Programs Offer
Prayer	27.17	52.17	10.17
Music	17.12	19.57	13.56
Nutrition	15.98	80.43	59.32
Chiropractic	12.56	23.91	27.12
Massage	12.10	39.13	61.02
Meditation	9.82	50.00	33.90
Mind/Body	9.82	32.61	50.85
Psychology	9.59	89.13	6.78
Yoga	7.76	17.39	27.12
Herbs	6.16	30.43	59.32
Reflexology	5.48	23.91	37.29
Acupuncture	5.02	56.52	35.59
Reiki	4.57	17.39	42.37
Homeopathic	4.34	26.09	40.68
Chinese Medicine	3.20	13.04	35.59
Naturopathy	1.60	15.22	16.95
Ayurveda	1.14	15.22	13.56

surveyed thought acupuncture (51 percent) was efficacious; 53 percent thought chiropractic was a valid approach for certain conditions; and 48 percent felt massage was useful. Fewer physicians (26 percent) thought homeopathy might be effective, and still fewer (13 percent) thought herbal approaches might work for their patients.

This literature review seems to indicate that significant numbers of physicians refer to or practice these five forms (acupuncture, chiropractic, homeopathy, herbal medicine, and massage) of CAM and that many physicians consider these therapies effective.

This book's survey asked thirty-five physicians about their use of and ideas pertaining to CAM. Thirty-five physicians of the 438 surveyed patients responded, including eleven medical doctors, ten doctors of osteopathy, three specialists, and nine residents (two others did not indicate their degrees). All the physicians indicated treating a wide variety of ailments. All indicated that they prescribed medications.

Significant numbers also indicated that they prescribed multi-vitamins and calcium, with more than one physician also prescribing Vitamins B, C, D, E, and folic acid. The number of physicians that prescribed herbals was barely significant (nine physicians). As mentioned, St. John's wort was most prescribed, but more than one physician also prescribed ginkgo biloba and goldenseal. The author speculates that ginkgo biloba was prescribed due to its popularity and press coverage as an aid to circulation and memory improvement, and that goldenseal was prescribed as an expectorant (the study was conducted in April at the end of a Northeastern, U.S. winter—i.e., during cold season). It is again worth noting that physicians classified glucosamine and chondroitin as herbal supplements and both were prescribed by more than one physician.

Physicians most often recommended the purchase of supplements at the pharmacy, but almost the same number recommended their purchase at health food stores. Grocery stores were not recommended as a place of purchase at the same rate that patients purchased them there, making another argument for convenience as being the main reason that patients pick up their supplements at supermarkets.

Significant numbers of physicians refer to the CAM practices of psychology, nutrition, pastoral counseling, and prayer (equal to psychology and nutrition when combined), and massage and acupuncture. Table 2.2 shows these referrals in reference to patient interests. The most striking difference is a seemingly high physician interest in acupuncture (more than 56 percent) with relatively low public interest in the practice (5 percent). This most likely indicates the growing conventional medical acceptance of acupuncture in the United States, at the same time that a cultural aversion to being stuck with needles exists among the general public.

As previously mentioned, physicians claimed that they learned about CAM from continuing education classes, or directly from practitioners of various modalities. They share the public's number-one mode of learning about CAM from practitioners themselves, but are also trusting of learning from other medical doctors. Although not a significant percentage, the media did appear third on the list of preferred learning methods.

COMPLEMENTARY AND ALTERNATIVE CLINICS

The CAM clinic survey was a mail survey of holistic health practitioners. Not all persons asked to participate responded. Four hundred surveys were mailed: 254 were to directory listings of holistic practitioners in Pennsylvania and Florida, 130 were to the top hospitals in the United States as chosen by *U.S. News & World Report* for 2000, and sixteen were CAM practices found on the Internet. Fifty-nine CAM businesses in Pennsylvania and Florida responded to the survey. A count of nine or 15.53 percent was considered statistically significant.

The group of greatest response was those with holistic directory listings in Pennsylvania. This may have been due to the author's location in Pennsylvania and the personalized approach (hand delivering surveys to all the patient and physician respondents by a person known to them created nearly 100 percent participation). Only two of 130 hospitals responded. Many of the surveys to hospitals were returned because the name of the CAM-related person at the hospital was unavailable, and most hospitals will not deliver mail that is not addressed to a specific person or department. Many of these surveys were returned with the names crossed off, blacked out, or scribbled out so violently that the pen marks tore through the envelopes. St. Luke's Hospital of Bethlehem, Pennsylvania, responded by e-mail explaining that there was no CAM at St. Luke's, and expressing incredulity that anyone should think so (St. Luke's has an award-winning pastoral care program operated by an acquaintance of the author). It also offers massage, yoga, and tai chi classes, but without central coordination. One suggested conclusion regarding the poor hospital response is that hospitals have large impersonal structures which are difficult to penetrate, in which one department is unaware of the existence of another. It is also possible that many staff members at these institutions harbor hostile attitudes toward CAM (see discussions of camps of thought in Chapter 1), despite the fact that CAM programs *do* operate at their institutions.

In February of 2001, the American Hospital Association reported that one of their surveys discerned that 500 hospitals had CAM programs, but they were unable to provide contact names for those programs. Time and expense, rather than lack of desire, prohibited further outreach to hospitals. The hospital's structures and administrative attitudes prevented their being a significant part of this survey.

The annual gross income of survey respondents was reported by not quite two-thirds (64 percent), but in significant enough numbers to conclude that operating a business offering CAM modalities is a viable devotion, earning full-time practitioners at least a livable wage. Of all respondents, 63 percent earned between $25,000 and $100,000 per year, with a mean income of $135,000. The average number of practitioners at businesses was four. Most practitioners (59 percent) indicated collaboration among practitioners and modalities, but a significant number did not do this formally. It is a recommendation of this work that CAM practices develop formal collaboration procedures to coordinate assessment and health practice plans.

Hourly rates for services ranged from $15 to $360 per hour, with an average of $77.75. Clearly no standard exists for CAM modality reimbursement. Some practitioners structure their practices with multiple clients waiting and less than an hour spent with each patient. Other practitioners spend large amounts of time with each client for small per-hour reimbursement rates.

A significant number of practices reported the regular use of sixteen different modalities: in order of use, they were massage, herbs, diet/nutrition, vitamins, Reiki, homeopathy, reflexology, Chinese medicine, meditation, chiropractic, yoga, therapeutic touch, nutraceuticals, electromagnetism, chi gung (or qi gong), and naturopathy (see Appendix C). It is very important to note that this was a survey of holistic health practitioners and not chiropractors, who are classified as another Standard Industrial Code (SIC) in directory listings and were not specifically surveyed here. Even so, many of the individual practitioners were chiropractors, and chiropractic made a strong showing as a CAM modality, despite its established strength in the United States under its own SIC classification. This means that chiropractors are open to and utilize many other types of CAM. This probably indicates not only the embrace of CAM by chiropractors but also the understanding of chiropractic's limitations as a complete medical system. However, one respondent disagreed with the classification of chiropractic as a body-based or manipulative modality and said it should be considered an alternative medical system. Body-based manipulation practices were reported as the number-one CAM offering by respondents. When adjusted for the fact that prayer, music, and psychology services are not offered to a great degree by these businesses, the interest of patients and the CAM clinic's offerings do correspond. CAM practices would be well advised, however, to note patient interests in prayer, pastoral counseling, and psychology, but especially in music and art therapy. It should be the role of CAM health plans to show how these practices integrate into a complete lifestyle plan.

CAM programs do not indicate that they work with their clients' primary care physicians. This is unfortunate, because physicians indicate that they most desire to learn about CAM from these practitioners. Only one CAM program respondent indicated that most of the program's referrals came from physicians. There is a relationship among physicians, CAM practitioners, and patients that is just waiting to happen, especially as indicated by physicians in residencies.

Most of the patients seen at CAM clinics came from word-of-mouth growth of these businesses (83 percent). Other ways of gaining clients (advertising and referral from other sources) were reported in insignificant numbers. It therefore stands to reason that the CAM businesses surveyed have already found a formula for some success based on what clients desire. None of the businesses reported constructing their practices through studying their clients. When the top three reasons for offering various modalities were ranked, CAM clinics reported that (1) it was their personal choice to do so, as the business owner, (2) it had proven conventional scientific efficacy, (3) it was safe for the client, and (4) it had a relaxing quality. No other reasons were significantly reported. The reasons to offer CAM to the public could be based on the rate and types of illness reported by those interested in CAM. It was not surprising to find that those interested in CAM were 5 percent more likely to be suffering from illness, but it is also interesting to compare the illnesses reported by those interested in CAM. Table 2.3 illustrates this. It would be wise for any CAM clinic to offer modalities aimed at alleviating these conditions.

It may be impressive that CAM practices have grown and prospered almost exclusively through word of mouth, but it also stands to reason that CAM businesses should seek to increase their exposure

TABLE 2.3. Greater Likeliness of Interest in CAM by Those Suffering from Illness (Percentage)

Illness	Interested	Not Interested	Percent More Likely to Be Interested
Overweight	36.73	26.89	9.84
Headaches	25.22	15.57	9.66
Anxiety	25.22	16.98	8.24
Allergy	22.12	13.21	8.92
Fatigue	16.81	8.96	7.85
High Blood Pressure	16.37	16.98	−0.61
Sinusitis	13.72	5.19	8.53
Arthritis	13.72	6.60	7.11
Asthma	13.27	8.96	4.31
Interpersonal Relations	9.73	4.72	5.02
High Cholesterol	9.29	7.55	1.74
Heart	8.85	6.60	2.25
Irritable Bowel	7.96	1.42	6.55
Diabetes	7.52	5.19	2.33
Attention Deficit	2.21	1.89	0.33
Osteoporosis	2.21	1.89	0.33
Cancer	1.33	0.47	0.86
Fibromyalgia	0.44	0.47	−0.03

and education of both the public and medical personnel by (1) advertising, (2) creating relationships with other practitioners and the medical community for referrals, and (3) offering seminars.

The survey did not ask what practitioners in CAM clinics considered an appropriate education, nor did it ask which modalities should and should not require licensing. The way CAM businesses select practitioners and how they should select them is a complicated question that will be discussed in greater depth in Chapter 3. CAM business operators rank their own personal choice highest in how they selected practitioners, followed by required licensing, and then appropriate education. This is strong evidence that despite the desire for objective qualifications, selection of practitioners is subjective.

Most CAM businesses reported that they operated as for-profit businesses (58 percent). Significant numbers reported that they were "loosely structured with practitioners paying rent" (32 percent), and that they were supervised by a medical or osteopathic doctor (17 percent).

CAM practices identified verbal feedback (90 percent) as their number-one source of knowledge for patient satisfaction. Fifty-four percent reported the continued growth of their business as evidence that patients were satisfied. Only fourteen (24 percent) resorted to a formal written survey for knowledge of patient satisfaction. CAM businesses would be well advised to make more formal assessments of patient satisfaction. It is understandable that CAM practices did not make formal assessments of the effectiveness of their modalities, as research for effectiveness is not usually within the scope of private practices that directly serve patients. Still, CAM practices considered verbal feedback and the continued growth of their businesses as being indicators for modality effectiveness. It is reasonable to deduce that patients consider they are deriving benefit from the modalities if they are both returning for services and recommending the services to friends and family. One respondent remarked that the question about ascertaining patient satisfaction and the effectiveness of services "were the same question." This was not the intent, however. Statistically demonstrable efficacy would not entail the same type of study as patient satisfaction. Lab indicators would have to be chosen for effectiveness (i.e., sustained drop in blood pressure for meditation as an intervention in its treatment). Although patients may be satisfied with the service, the desired health effect may not have been achieved. Chapter 1 of this work lists several studies of effectiveness of these modalities for particular health conditions.

Sixty-eight percent of the CAM clinic respondents follow up with patients by scheduling another appointment, while 41 percent reported making a phone call for follow-up. It was not an expected outcome of this survey to find this level of follow-up, especially for the busier clinics reporting high incomes. All but one of the ten respondents reporting higher-than-average income claimed that they used both the scheduling of appointments and phone calls to follow up with clients. These methods may indicate the most important type of marketing a CAM practice can do to ensure success. Many conventional medical practices schedule follow-up visits for various conditions, but how many physicians or employees of physicians make calls to see how their patients are doing?

Product Sales

The sale of products to clients is another important consideration for CAM practices. The programs surveyed were not classified as retail outlets, yet 70 percent sold products. Of those practices with incomes above average, all but one sold products, and seven of these ten programs reported more than 10 percent of their income from product sales, with three reporting that 70 to 80 percent of their income was from product sales. Of those reporting a percentage of income for product sales, the average amount of income from these sales was 21 percent—a significant amount, especially for nonretail businesses.

The sale of products remains controversial in CAM practices, although many conventional medical practices now offer on-site prescription services. Some practitioners identify the sale of products with "profiteering" and believe it subtracts from the equation of healing. Most, however, do not feel this way and readily offer products for sale. The most popular reported product sales in order (see Appendix C) are (1) nutritional supplements, (2) herbs, and (3) homeopathic medicines. It is important to note that these are all available in easy-to-take pill, powder, and tincture forms, and once again demonstrates the public's desire for a quick fix. Compact discs and tapes ranked significantly, but the opportunity to satisfy the public interest expressed in the patient survey for music and art therapy should be taken advantage of in educating patients how to specifically use music, artwork, videos, and musical instruments in their health care plans.

Insurance

Three questions on the survey asked specifically about insurance or third-party reimbursement for services. A fourth question asked what practitioners thought was the biggest impediment to the growth of CAM. The largest percentage (39 percent) believed that the inability to accept insurance was the biggest impediment with a little more than half of that (22 percent) placing public confusion over CAM in a distant second place. Thirty-five respondents (59 percent) said that they did accept insurance payments. The only significant areas that were reported to accept insurance were chiropractic and massage (see Appendix C). It was very surprising to find that at least one program claimed to also accept insurance for Chinese medicine (presumably acupuncture), diet and nutrition, homeopathy, biofeedback, herbs, therapeutic touch, osteopathic manipulation, and nutraceuticals. Even chi gung, reflexology, Reiki, and tai chi were listed as having one practitioner who accepted insurance reimbursement. Although a follow-up to this survey is not immediately planned, asking these practitioners how they managed to utilize third-party reimbursement for these practices might assist in extending CAM practices' ability to charge third parties for reimbursement. When asked to rank on a scale of one to ten the importance of their ability to accept insurance in their ability to offer CAM, respondents' answers covered the gamut of one to ten. Thirty-six (61 percent) said it was of greater than average (5 on the scale) importance with an average ascribed importance of 6.49 percent on the scale of one to ten. Perhaps most significantly, fourteen (24 percent) said it was of greatest importance (10 on the scale).

CONCLUSION

This chapter summarizes the original research done by the author for the intention of making recommendations regarding the structure of a health clinic. Subsequent chapters will report recommendations for choosing modalities and on design and structure of complementary and alternative medicine clinics.

Chapter 3

Choosing Modalities for a Clinic

The first chapter of this book deals with the classifications (domains) of CAM and a description of some of the modalities available in each one. CAM in the United States today is, without a doubt, a confusing labyrinth of options. Some of these modalities are new introductions of the techniques of other cultures, the revival of ancient traditions, or the "modality du jour" in keeping with the latest trends or fads. To make matters worse, some offerings combine a trendy approach with ancient tradition in a haphazard fashion. Yoga is not a lifestyle direction in the United States, but a weekly (or perhaps daily) workout routine. A type of yoga meant for warriors in ancient India was made into something called "power yoga" to satisfy our aggressive American appetites. It has been heralded as proof that yoga is not just for "women and wimps." This plays on stereotypical views of yoga, women, and the Western sacrilege of being nonaggressive in an almost nasty way. At its very best, practicing power yoga in this way may get people to exercise who may otherwise have stayed sedentary. At its worst, it bastardizes yoga to the point of being unrecognizable, in a similar way that processing and bleaching flour will give us a quicker carbohydrate buzz but avoids the inconveniences (and benefits) of fiber. Finally, in Chinese taoist terms, it speaks of our belief that only the yang (or masculine principle) is good, and that balance of yin (or female principle) and yang is somehow undesirable.

Let there be no mistake. The CAM revolution in medicine is due to the need to balance medicine by bringing back the slower, more introspective yin principles to health. Taking balanced forms of lifestyle adaptations and making them more palatable to a speedy, aggressive culture will not produce the desired effect. The first consideration in choosing *complementary* modalities for a clinic is to offer things that are not offered at the offices of conventional medical doctors and in hospitals. Some of those considerations are as follows:

1. Take time with patients, allowing them to gain introspection.
2. Relax and slow the pace of patients, centering them in the present.
3. Offer thoughtful expansion on *alternatives* available, engaging patients to think for themselves, study the possibilities, and listen to an inner voice in choosing modalities *and* making decisions concerning conventional treatment.

When considering the scientific efficacy of modalities, make no mistake: there are separate camps when considering various options. Whether or not clear research verifies the effectiveness of homeopathy is something of *bitter* controversy. It is bitter, because these disagreements in the scientific community are emotional battles, fought by people with different beliefs, with one side merely scoffing at the other, or misleading the public by crying fouls such as fraud and even insanity. Whether you are a self-proclaimed shaman who channels angels to new-age music, or the wizened chief of surgery of a huge hospital who considers all of CAM to be "snake oil," know that no black-and-white issues exist in medicine, research, science, or metaphysics. Your patients and clients are in the gray area, where reality is firmly located, and together you are really just poking about seeing what things will help and what will not. To put it succinctly, a large dose of humility is required in offering health care options to the public.

Unfortunately, to make it all worse, some people in conventional medicine and in CAM have no problem with misleading the public; they do so believing it is for the public's own good. Therefore, it is essential that all practitioners and clinics offer complete information to the public about their modalities. For example, the FDA requirement that drugs be proven safe and effective is a bastion of false security, because it suggests that absolute proof exists. It is not usually shared with patients the fact that some widely used medications have effectiveness rates that are only marginally within the framework of statistical significance for effectiveness. Studies that seem to have shown 100 percent effectiveness of any treatment always lose such perfection as the drug is further studied and its long-range effects and side effects are learned. Assume that your patients (1) are intelligent and wise enough to make their own decisions and that they *must* get the best information to do this and (2) know more about their health than you do, because it is *their* personal mind, body, and spirit. The trick is getting enough information from them, so you can make decisions together (see the section on assessment in Chapter 4, and assessment tools in Appendix D).

The ideal CAM clinic works in conjunction with a personal or family physician. Surgery and drugs are not options that are to be thrown away in health care because of the camps of belief and interpretation of science. The family physician should be engaged as part of a team for the health care consumer's benefit, with the *health care consumer* making the final decision when disagreements occur. Even when physicians disagree with or are staunchly against CAM interventions, an educated client can listen to the reasons on both sides and make a mature decision. This is accomplished through the calming and centering of the health care consumer in the present (see Chapter 4).

CHOOSING MODALITIES

Use Chapter 1 as a guide in understanding the broad classifications of treatment types and selecting modalities for a clinic. All these modalities are reviewed in this section. The research in Chapter 2 outlines some differences in the interests and practices of physicians, patients, and clinics offering CAM modalities. After considering these differences, the following recommended modalities are presented in the order of interest and use as reported by clients. When structuring a clinic, however, give attention to the five domains and, when possible, offer many services or referrals that cover this broad range. These recommendations account for both the current practices and reported interest of the health care consumers and their physicians.

Spiritual Counseling and Prayer

Studies already cited and reported in *JAMA* show that the public is interested in CAM because it ascribes a relevance and importance to spiritual values and health. Western culture is far from devoid of the application of prayer and pastoral counseling to health. Patients and their families at hospitals have the option of contacting religious leaders from their churches, synagogues, and mosques, or consulting with staff from hospital pastoral care programs. Very few object to praying over patients, whether it is believed as a viable complement or not. Some more exotic or unusual folk beliefs and practices that are culturally appropriate for certain patients may be frowned on at certain hospitals but should be considered powerful complements to treatment.

When offering complementary and alternative options, ask questions about the patients' spiritual practices and beliefs to ascertain both possible complements to care and areas lacking in balance in their lives. Caution must be exercised in this regard: independent CAM clinics are least versed in offering these interventions, but patients are extremely interested in them. Still, offense may be taken by a patient because of sudden prodding for his or her spiritual practices. After all, spiritual health is the ultimate expression of holism, and many of our physical and psychological foibles are obstacles (or opportunities!) that are strewn on the path to great personal and spiritual growth. Many patients are not cognitively ready to deal with this: it is why they have become physically ill in the first place. In asking what methods will work best for a particular patient, it must be determined if the patient already has a good relationship with a member of his or her own traditional or chosen faith community. If the patient has no relationship, it is very strongly recommended that some practice be adopted to develop a spiritual life. This may be as simple as beginning a practice in meditation or yoga, and/or increasing awareness through guided meditation. It might also mean some counseling sessions with family clergy, or the inclusion of family prayer into their lives. At any rate, these are small steps, with the idea that the ultimate goal of holistic health is the spiritual growth of the individual. In many cases, the message is received loud and clear after a crisis by patients when, for example, they have a heart attack, survive surgery, then decide to learn meditation in order to slow themselves down and be able to spend more time with loved ones. Many people seek CAM and perhaps most seek CAM because they are already taking the next step in their own spiritual development. This reality makes the role of programs offering CAM especially important. Health care consumers may come wanting to take a next step, but they are not sure what this should be and are seeking guidance. Interviewing individuals at an initial assessment will uncover some of these spiritual needs and may suggest directions for the individuals to travel.

Music and Art Therapy

One of the small surprises in the clinic survey was a strong interest expressed in the use of music and art to intervene in ill health and promote well-being. Music, art, dance, rhythm, and movement can be used effectively for some patients. Some of these activities can be offered as group activities—dancing, drumming, painting, and sculpting, to mention a few. Shyer persons can have one-on-one treatment sessions with music and art therapists. Many modalities such as dance, yoga, massage, and hypnosis incorporate the use of music. CAM clinics can offer the music that they use in their modalities for sale for patients' personal use. Associating a particular piece of music with relaxation is like having a favorite chair or comfortable spot at home; as soon as one approaches this space, one begins to relax in memory and expectation of positive results. It would be difficult to argue that individuals can have too many soothing and healing things in their environment.

Nutrition

Nutritional counseling can be done by dietitians or other holistic health counselors. CAM offers a significant array of theory and practice in diet, nutrition, and digestion. Some of these theories conflict with one another. It may be important for someone who is trained in determining nutritional deficiencies, such as a naturopathic physician, to examine and test patients for such deficiencies. At times, only a conventional medical doctor can order the multiple tests required to determine deficiencies. It is recommended that persons suffering from health difficulties adopt diets and eating habits based on their needs, and that they consider appropriate supplementation in order to get the best nutrition. CAM clinics can also offer for sale to their clients the herbs and supplements that they recommend and, according to the survey, a majority of programs do.

Body-Based/Manipulation Interventions

It is next recommended to offer some services within the body-based/manipulation therapies domain. Patients report chiropractic and massage as interests. It may not be necessary to have a chiropractor at a CAM clinic due to the availability of private chiropractic offices, but it is recommended that a chiropractor work together with all professionals engaged in improving the health of an individual. Massage is recommended for many conditions, either as a direct intervention for pain, injury, or discomfort, or for increasing relaxation and improving the overall well-being of a patient. The relaxation response is useful in reducing blood pressure, anxiety, and depression, and in improving immune function.

Mind/Body Interventions: Yoga, Tai Chi, Chi Gung, Meditation, and Holistic Psychology

Patients show a substantial interest in practices within the realm of the mind/body domain, with over 35 percent saying they are interested in or already using these modalities. Patients deserve to know that they can participate in their own care by using their minds on many different levels. Guided meditation calms and centers patients so that they can focus on their own health needs. Yoga, tai chi, and qi gong increase awareness of coordination of body signals and functions. Biofeedback techniques control physiological markers such as blood pressure. Hypnosis and neurolinguistic programming (a technique that uses self-repetition of short phrases to produce a desired effect on one's body) can also help to create better health habits. The choices in mind/body therapies are many. The client's needs and amount of time available are the main considerations in creating a plan that is considered realistic, but at least one of these techniques that help draw the patient into the present should be considered.

Herbs

Both clients and physicians expressed a strong interest in herbs, with 12 percent of clients reporting that they use herbs and 26 percent of physicians reporting that they prescribe them. Although this method of intervention is one of the more popular, it remains an area fraught with controversy. Often, neither patients nor physicians have the expertise required to prescribe herbs.

Health food stores are filled with herbs, and often the sales are linked to the latest media exposure of a particular herb, or to someone coming in because a friend told him or her a certain herb was effective for a particular ill, or because they used an herb reference book in a store to "look up" a quick prescription. Sometimes these methods may work, and when the prescribed herb is a food herb, such as ginger or garlic, there is perhaps no harm or ill effect, and benefit can be gained. Medicinal herbs, however, work more like prescription medications (it is important to remember that they *were* the prescriptive medicines for centuries). What medical doctors are no longer versed in, the herbalist still is, thus keeping the tradition alive. Many persons may be knowledgeable about herbs, but only three types are likely to understand the intricacies of potency, herbal blends, and dosage. One would be a person from a family with an oral tradition handed down through generations, another would be a naturopathic physician, and the most formally trained in this particular craft would be a person who has the American Herbalists Guild (AHG) degree. Guild titles from other countries would also be knowledgeable, as would practitioners of Ayurvedic, Tibetan, Chinese, and other systems of indigenous medicine.

Acupuncture

This area is of high interest to physicians, but one of the lowest areas of interest for patients (perhaps because of our limited cultural acceptance of piercing needles through the skin). This modality, in most places, can be practiced only by a certified person (certification requirements defined by the state) and under the supervision of a physician. This proscription limits the CAM practices able to offer acupuncture, but of course it is a strong complement for pain relief, and is likely to have many more benefits that are farther-reaching.

Reiki and Therapeutic Touch

These modalities are classified in the energy/metaphysical domain. The controversy concerning TT is discussed in Chapter 1. Although an insignificant number of patients (1.14 percent) said that they used Reiki, three times as many expressed interest in learning more about it, which is significant. It is important to note that patients were slightly (although insignificantly) more interested in acupuncture than Reiki. One physician claimed to refer patients to practitioners of Reiki, but no physicians expressed interest in learning more about it. This indicates an increasing interest by the public in the modality, but disagreement in the medical community as to its usefulness, one of the true hallmarks of CAM.

This domain is outside the realm of the physical sciences, even though, as discussed regarding prayer, its effectiveness can be discerned. Clearly, these modalities have an incredible safety rate, and a well-reported relaxation benefit, making the controversy of little concern. Practitioners of TT are nurses, although others could be trained in it. Reiki practitioners are trained through what is essentially an oral tradition of Reiki, where training and certification can be bestowed by persons who have completed a higher level of training. This training process is not monitored by any organization, although recommendations of how the training should proceed are made by the International Center for Reiki Training in Southfield, Michigan. As always, these modalities are a concern only when they are touted as a total alternative with the ability to cure, rather than as a complementary therapy.

Homeopathy

Homeopathy is insignificantly reported as used by or of interest to physicians. A small but significant number (3.42 percent) of patients expressed a desire to learn more about it. Less than 1 percent of patients reported using homeopathy. The persons qualified to prescribe homeopathy are the few medical doctors who still use it, naturopathic physicians, and persons well studied in the field. Because homeopathic remedies have minute or mere "energy signature" contents of a mother substance, its risks are negligible. Arguably, those who may successfully practice the art can include persons other than licensed or degreed professionals, because of homeopathy's intricate and well-developed history-taking procedure, and the materia medica of homeopathic remedies is based on the results of this history taking. In other words, homeopathy relies less on education, intuition, and experience more than does the prescription of pharmaceuticals. It would not be fair, however, to say that experience is not necessary in the practice of homeopathy, as the question of potency and frequency of dosage is best left to an experienced practitioner, most likely to be either a naturopath or medical doctor.

GETTING THE WORD OUT

Most new programs will not want to start offering all the modalities listed. It is recommended to start at the top of the list with the first one, two, or three in order to build clientele and interest. It is also recommended that a local clinic gauge interest by surveying their patients or community members, as well as by offering seminars to groups. It is important to emphasize outreach by choosing groups to present to off site, rather than trying to attract crowds to seminars at the clinic. A significant amount of time and expense for promotion could be saved by calling and working directly with local social service and disease-specific programs. Civic groups, health food stores and cooperatives, and the health and social welfare committees of large area religious groups might also be contacted.

Large practices with a significant number of clients and practices with retail operations that get foot traffic can attempt to sign up people for classes at their location, if the facility permits.

"Tabling" (placing a table with information on services) at health care events and health fairs is often considered a good way to attract interest. These events usually end up promoting a concept in general and a few will return to your practice because of such exposure. Some practices, such as massage and other body-based techniques, may be an exception to this, as direct service can be rendered as a short sampling and a business card can be passed to the person with a coupon recommending that they call for a full hour at a discounted price, if they enjoyed the sample. The practitioners must realize, of course, that this is a long day of "free" work for a limited return. A homeopath would have little success with such an approach, and offering a general talk would elicit little direct return. Still, it is highly recommended to engage in *all these types of exposure* at least twice a year, despite the seemingly small return.

QUALIFICATIONS OF PRACTITIONERS

Practitioner qualification is a difficult question, and one given to much debate. If a modality such as massage or naturopathy requires licensing in a particular state, little question arises about who is qualified to perform that modality. For this reason alone this book recommends that all the modalities work toward the concept of licensing or state-level recognition of certification for each modality. Professional organizations within CAM have set up certification examinations, but sometimes these organizations oppose one another within the same field. This book will not argue these points, because although these groups claim quality and protection of the public on the surface, they are political activists in the end, trying to claim turf over one group or another.

Still, there must be some way to assure that persons performing health interventions have been trained properly and are conducting reasonably safe practices. Following is a summary of possibilities for qualifications organized by the five domains.

Alternative Medical Systems

To determine proper qualifications of practitioners, established schools from the countries and cultures where various alternative medical systems originate should be consulted as to whether the practitioners in question have received satisfactory training. Examples of this would include consulting Chinese schools of medicine or Indian schools of Ayurveda, and requesting diploma or transcript information on its qualified graduates. Determining the credentials of a foreign school could include reviewing length of existence, number of graduates, and especially the activities of its graduates. These qualified persons could in turn be the ones doing the training in the United States.

This credential information would then flow to those CAM professional organizations setting up educational programs (or registering current ones) and applying for proper accreditation from the regional body recognized by the U.S. Department of Education (DOE). The NIH's National Center for Complementary and Alternative Medicine (NCCAM) could keep a registry of such organizations, their educational programs, and their status for accreditation.

Licensing exams could be created by the CAM professional organizations and submitted to various state commissions set up to approve and write licensing exams and procedures.

This is all a tedious process—note the previously mentioned debacle of naturopathy where an insufficient number of schools have been able to garner accreditation, multiple organizations have cropped up in the vacuum within the practice to claim they are such accrediting bodies; few states have licensing for naturopathy and confusion reigns supreme.

If there is a serious desire in the current U.S. government administration to bring the most effective CAM to U.S. citizens in a way that requires the highest quality practitioners, NCCAM will need to open an office which will be the authority that formally recognizes the national organizations that will do this work. A formal application process should be established by the office which might take a period of two to five years, and then decisions should be made on which organizations are recognized for any given discipline. One single organization could dare to become the National Complementary and Alternative Medical Association, but quality control for vast traditions such as Chinese medicine and Ayurveda are best left to unique organizations.

Mind/Body Interventions

This work uses a modified form of NCCAM's classifications specifically so that the domains can be used to more clearly focus on issues of practitioner qualifications. Methods such as prayer have been relegated to the energy/metaphysical classification so that they may enjoy the legal status they have always had.

In the domain of mind/body interventions, for example, biofeedback is a seldom-mentioned mind/body technique with some impressive research. However, licensing and instrument calibration requirements have made it prohibitively expensive and have all but killed it. Caution is advised in developing policies that will cause this to happen to effective interventions that could help thousands.

Since meditation is self-practiced and part of long-standing Eastern intellectual and mystical traditions it does not seem that such rigorous attention needs to be applied to it. Hypnosis and art and music therapy, however, may need to have the same system applied to its schools and national organization as the process discussed under alternative medical systems.

Biologically Based Therapies

Practitioners of alternative medical systems recommend many biologically based therapies. The FDA should look at standards for potency (not necessarily pharmaceutical content perfection) and minimum dosage for efficacy, as well as labeling requirements for consumers.

Body-Based Manipulation Therapies

Massage is well on its way to the level of organization achieved by nursing or the AMA. Several states already have licensing; use these as models for the rest of the country. Chiropractic has completed this licensing process, as has osteopathy, which is now recognized on par with traditional medicine. This domain seems to be moving in a definite direction and may need little assistance, but would benefit from a NCCAM organizational accrediting office.

Energy/Metaphysical Therapies

NCCAM classifies magnetic, electricity, and other detectable fields and energies in this domain, but a similar approach should be made to these interventions as those listed in the Biologically Based Interventions section. It is hoped that the FDA could be convinced to determine and label the strength of shoe magnets, for example.

As for the undetectable and metaphysical energies present in such therapies as prayer, Reiki, TT, and shamanism, these are in the same realm as religious traditions and the same exemptions applied to clergy in their ministry to the sick should be applied to these practitioners.

CONCLUSION: APPLYING MULTIPLE CRITERIA TO CHOOSING MODALITIES

Despite these accreditation recommendations, which hold no promise for resolving issues of qualifications anytime soon, CAM programs operate throughout the United States. Most successful CAM programs surveyed were supervised by physicians, chiropractors, or nurse practitioners, and they reported that the number-one reason (54 percent) for choosing a practitioner was "personal choice." In other words, the industry currently operates a step away from licensing of modalities, by having licensed professionals handpick practitioners of these modalities for their patients. What criteria did they use to select them? Fifty-one percent said licensing, if required; 41 percent said appropriate education, presumably determined by them with the practitioners presenting their credentials; 25 percent said professional affiliation (such as membership in the American Massage Therapy Association); 18 percent said that clients had recommended practitioners; and 17 percent said they were concerned with the number of years of experience held by CAM practitioners. Currently, the process is that of interview and presentation of qualifications: the process most typically followed for hiring in the United States. This form of assessing qualification for the performance of even complex tasks requiring extensive training has proven effective in businesses for hundreds of years, so it should not be discounted as a sound method that the public can feel reasonably assured will bring them a competent health care provider.

Whether you are a medical person, a businessperson or practitioner interested in setting up a CAM health program, or a patient looking for options and additions in health treatments, the task in choosing modalities is the same. You must digest the available information on safety and effectiveness (see Chapter 1) and determine whether the options are viable for cost reasons. You must then determine whether there are persons who can provide effective health care within these particular modalities. That there is significant interest in CAM is no longer in question. If you are a scientist, you know that no absolutes exist, and that scientific evidence merely reports for or against something. *You* must digest what this information is; reliance on other people's opinions is possible but not recommended. What is really being recommended here is that a patient *no longer be a patient,* having things "done to them" in matters of health. Patients must become clients; as clients, they should be informed consumers of health options. If they are to be successful, practitioners and CAM businesses must have a wide range of information available to their clients and learn how to work with their clients in helping them make the best health decisions.

Chapter 4

Clinic Design and Structure

Many approaches can be taken to the design and structure of a health care clinic, including incorporating the good aspects of traditional health care—at physician and chiropractor offices—with some of the more effective aspects of social services. These social service aspects include the concepts of wraparound services—multiple services that the patient needs—and peer support.

TRADITIONAL STRUCTURES

Traditionally, health care is structured either as a private consultation practice of a health professional (such as physician, osteopath, or chiropractor), or in a hospital setting. Recently, emergency clinics have also emerged as twenty-four-hour services that integrate the feel of the doctor's office with the convenience of walk-in service at any time of day. These operations often include pharmacy, lab, and some physical therapy components similar to a hospital.

Drawbacks of the traditional physician's office include long waits for brief services. Here a lack of careful history taking for illnesses occurs and symptoms are treated without seeking to solve root causes. This is compounded by the fact that each incidence of illness is treated as a separate occurrence unrelated to other illnesses and conditions that the health care consumer may be experiencing or has experienced in the past. The typical visit consists of the client *briefly* stating symptoms, after which the physician delivers a diagnosis and pulls out the prescription pad (after, perhaps, a brief reference to medical material). To be blunt, this environment would be a better description of how a psychic healer's office would operate, for one would have to be psychic to *always* correctly diagnose and treat so many cases in so little time. Only the annual physical with its accompanying lab tests delivers the type of health care that Western medicine intends. Unfortunately, it is once again the impatience of the health care consumers (and their lack of funds) that restricts the thorough exploration that lab tests can give in diagnosing illnesses. Since the conventional medical doctor is *not* psychic, nor does he or she pretend to be so, it is this vast science from which the doctor's craft springs. This science is the friend of the client in uncovering medical truth. Since the office approach of the medical doctor is not likely to change anytime soon, two pieces of advice are given to the client: (1) find a highly intuitive practitioner and (2) seek a thorough health program that (a) introduces the idea of healthy lifestyle, (b) helps with diagnosed illness, (c) explores the root causes to illness, and (d) works to prevent its return. It is into this vacuum listed as the second piece of advice that CAM steps.

The second point of comparison for traditional health programs in the United States is the hospital. This model draws together practitioners from various disciplines or specialties. In theory, this gives the health care consumer the advantage of coordinated care. In other words, internal medicine physicians, surgeons, disease specialists, nurses, nutritionists, psychologists, social workers, and physical therapists work together to heal the patient. Most hospitals also have a chaplain or a pastoral care program. Many hospitals may also have an integrative medicine program usually including massage, yoga, and meditation, but the hospital may offer these as open programs to individuals living in the community that the hospital serves rather than as integrative care to an admitted patient. No other organization in today's medical care structure than the hospital would be better equipped to integrate all the potent interventions CAM has to offer. However, what lacks are (1) a relaxation of the "camps of thought"—a mentality that keeps many CAM practices from the patient in the hospital setting, and (2) a consistent coordinated effort that will lead to a plan which will fully and accurately assess a patient, recommending lifestyle changes, and keeping the patient on track.

At their worst, hospitals are huge impersonal organizations that treat patients as numbers instead of people and whose environment of illness contributes to poor health rather than to healing. Not only is care not coordinated, but incorrect treatments are given to patients in mix-ups, heroic surgeries are fouled up, and patients receive medications that cause further complications. Indeed, the hospital in many instances has become a repository of botched medical intervention. Adverse drug reactions (ADRs) cost the health system an estimated $76.6 billion each year; 62 percent of those costs ($47.5 billion) are for hospitalizations. A meta-analysis of thirty-nine studies of hospitalization rates from ADRs found the average prevalence to be 6.7 percent of all admissions (Lazarou, Pomeranz, and Corey, 1998). The U.S. General Accounting Office (2000) estimated this same rate to be as high as 1,200 incidents per 100 admissions in nursing homes. In addition, in the outpatient setting an estimated 2 percent of outpatient prescriptions resulted in probable or definite adverse reactions; 61 percent of these ADRs require subsequent health visits. Finally, a study by the Physician Insurers Association of America showed that medication errors are the second most frequent physician malpractice claim (Ulrich, 1998).

The problems facing the true integration of CAM with conventional medicine still abound, although much progress has been made in the modalities accepted and offered to the community by hospitals. Many opportunities arise in light of this fact, for CAM practices to emerge by offering patients hope in integrated assessment and healthy lifestyle techniques. For this purpose, a theoretical model of the root causes of illness is offered as a guide to CAM clinics wishing to integrate techniques and focus on the care of their clients. The author's twenty-five years of nonprofit health experience have culminated in offering a clinic design that incorporates a blend of the health care and social service models, as well as a multidisciplinary assessment procedure aimed at thoroughness in care.

THEORETICAL MODEL OF ILLNESS

Figure 4.1 shows the causes and triggers of illness. The model separates illness causes from illness triggers, thus explaining why seemingly identical conditions may cause illness for some but not for others.

This model is also broken up into external (those influences from the outside of the patient) and internal factors. Further classifications show that physiological, psychological, spiritual, and social factors are present in the world both as external and internal influences. Self-explanatory in the way it is organized, the figure is offered here as the

Illness Causes —These are the factors that must be present to cause illness. There must be at least one internal and one external factor to cause illness. These should receive at least palliative treatment, counseling or social intervention, but may not be the main focus of treatment. Illness causes without a triggering factor *do not* proceed to a diagnosable illness.

Internal		External	
Physiological— Chemical imbalances, genetic predispositions, injury, organic damage.	*Psychological—* Past or childhood experiences.	*Physiological—* Exposure to pathogens, chemicals, sensitive and allergic substances.	*Psychosocial—* Daily stress factors. External psychological triggers are cultural or social in nature. Drug or sexual subcultures, peer-group pressure, etc.

Illness Triggers are the proverbial straws that break the camels' backs. They do not cause disorders themselves but trigger or precipitate them. They can also increase intensity and reoccurrence. In fact, if not dealt with, reoccurrence is likely. These triggers may become the main focus of treatment.

Internal		External	
Physiological— Weakened systems of the body: Digestive, cardiovascular, etc. These can be isolated and controlled through lifestyle factors.	*Psychospiritual—* The personal issues of the disorder which are issues that can be internally isolated, influenced, or controlled. These have to do with self-perception in relation to the world and/or to a spiritual life.	*Physiological—* Damage to the body caused by the exposure to pathogens, chemicals, allergens, and sensitive substances.	*Psychological—* Damage caused by repetitive behavior from daily stress, and cultural and social stresses.

Diagnosable Illness

FIGURE 4.1. Illness model showing the flow from causes to triggers of diagnosable illness.

philosophical and theoretical basis for the rest of this chapter concerning areas of assessment as well as clinic design and structure.

Illness causes can be equated with risk factors. The triggers for disease are those instances in which causative factors are set into an active disease state by a precipitating circumstance. This author's opinion is that the precipitating factor is psychospiritual in nature. For example, have you or anyone you have known ever come down with a severe cold just before an important date or event? This illness model considers the root causes and precipitating factors. The illness causes might be (1) an external pathogen, or rhinovirus, and (2) an internal inability of the immune system to ward it off. The illness triggers might be the fear or concern over the important date or event. Perhaps the worry caused the run-down condition that led to an insufficient immune response, but in the end it is the trigger (the worry and concern) that must be satisfactorily dealt with in order to reduce the number of colds suffered, and to reduce the cold's severity and the patient's susceptibility. This model may be simple when considered with this example, but if kept simple this differentiation between internal and external causes and triggers can assist in thorough assessment for even complicated illnesses. The CAM structure of the five domains allows CAM practitioners to apply treatments to these internal and external factors.

Assessment

As discussed, the assessment process takes into account the internal and external physiological, psychosocial, and psychospiritual causes and triggers of disease.

Physiological

Chemical imbalances, genetic predispositions, injury, organic damage, and nutritional deficiency are typical physiological problems. Assessment in this realm is done by those licensed to diagnose and treat physical illness. Lab tests are done where appropriate to discern any of these root causes or triggers. A CAM practitioner may suspect any of the above and recommend that the client approach his or her family physician to have tests done accordingly. Ideally, a CAM clinic has licensed physicians on its team; less ideally, a CAM health center can have a two-way relationship with their clients' physicians; and least ideally, a client can be the sole mode of communication between the two, creating some kind of communication, however uneasy. Physiological health problems can be suspected by any CAM practitioner through physical examination, and intuitive means. It is strongly recommended that such revelations be confirmed or denied through Western scientific testing methods.

Psychosocial/Psychospiritual

Similarly, diagnosis and treatment for psychological illnesses fall within the jurisdiction of licensed psychology professionals, but the psychological and psychospiritual or spiritual causes and triggers of illness fall somewhat in a gray area. These ideas are not (currently) a part of conventional treatments of illness. Guidance and probing is recommended to come from an experienced practitioner with a modality that discerns mind/body types (Chinese medicine, Ayurveda, homeopathy, and the California school of Louise Hay as described in works such as *You Can Heal Your Life* [1987], to name four).

The assessment instrument in Appendix D flows into completing the assessment by determining and listing the internal and external features of illness. A health plan is then written after the patient has reviewed, understands, and agrees to the assessment.

CLINIC DESIGN AND STRUCTURE

Figure 4.2 shows the structure and flow of a CAM health clinic. This model follows a social-services concept for health care.

Client Intake

Practitioners working together can take turns or determine another method for selecting who shall work as the intake person. This person can use their practice discipline (such as Ayurveda, Chinese medicine, or naturopathy) as the first line of intervention. It is recommended that one of the disciplines from the domain of alternative medical systems, or an MD, DO, DC, or nurse practitioner do the client intake and assessment. The health assessment tools instrument (Appendix D) shows the author's thorough health assessment rou-

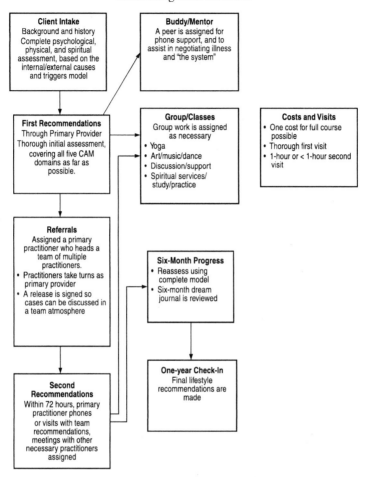

FIGURE 4.2. Model for a multidisciplinary holistic health clinic.

tine, which combines conventional, medical, Ayurvedic, psychological, and social-service models. *It is paramount that all the necessary time should be taken to complete this assessment.* Parts of it can be made into a questionnaire that can be mailed to the client before an appointment so that he or she can spend the time to be thorough, but the practitioner *must* review and *comprehend* the material and evaluate it with the client, asking questions of the client as necessary to clarify his or her understanding of the material.

The health assessment in Appendix A is a lengthy survey aimed at uncovering problems in the physiological, psychological, social, and spiritual realms. Clients can receive the questionnaire by mail, or perhaps complete it on the Internet if posted. In any case, they should be encouraged to take the time that they require to answer the questions thoroughly. The practitioner can then finish the survey as part of the first appointment. A concentrated and thorough review of the health assessment form along with the information from an initial meeting are required to develop initial recommendations. One technique that may be useful is that some suggestions can be made at the initial intake, with more to be faxed, mailed, e-mailed, or phoned to the client at a prescribed time after the practitioner has made a thorough review of the intake. It may seem irregular to the client, but when it is explained that this process encourages quality and thoroughness, it is believed that this new approach will be considered preferable. Often, individuals seeking CAM assistance have already visited many different doctors looking for answers, and have been suffering problems for months and even years. An additional waiting period will seem minimal for a more complete assessment.

The following section refers to the health assessment in Appendix D by question number, and serves as the procedure for health care practitioners. Figure 4.3 shows a sample of a possible completed health plan for a client developed from the assessment. Rather than explain each question, it is assumed that professional health care practitioners will be familiar with the reasons for collecting and using such data to arrive at justifiable conclusions.

1. Always follow up to ensure that the client truly suffers from a prediagnosed condition. Although diplomacy methods are beyond the scope of this work, take care to not insult either the client or his or her diagnosing practitioner.
2. Check questions 2, 3, 4, and 5 for possible adverse reactions among medications. It is important to note this is inclusive of caffeine, alcohol, tobacco, and other drug (illegal) interactions. It takes a while to check this and it is best not to keep a client waiting. Although a Web site, such as <www.drugchecker. drkoop.com> can be useful, never blindly enter drug names looking for interactions; rather, check for interactions with drug *types* and similar substances. Practitioners who can assess the

client's constitutional type will recognize individual foods and substances, as well as interactions, that might aggravate particular mind/body types.

7. Give special attention to the words the client uses to describe her or his condition and for underlying emotional (or lack of emotional) reaction. In addition to being aware of overly stoic or emotional descriptions in answer to this question, check the tone of voice of the client for repression, fear, anger, and depression. Your client knows his or her own body, so pay attention to the client, both verbally and nonverbally!

9. Use questions 7, 9, and 10 as different ways of revealing more about the client, but question 9 may raise some of the frustrations clients have had in receiving complete or satisfactory health services.

11. Use question 11 in writing the client health plan. The plan will be meaningful only if it incorporates client goals. At the seventy-two-hour follow-up, the practitioner should clarify how each recommended plan to reduce the risk factors is in line with the client's goals.

13. The illness chart presents opportunities to express health problems in various ways to elicit information.

21. Use this chart to write the psychological and social factors into the health plan, trying to move all twenty-four items toward the "Always" answer.

22. Questions 22 and 23 deal with the spiritual and metaphysical realm. Encourage all clients to find a way in which to express their spiritual natures. Often this spiritual expression is achieved by finding the right mix of cultural appropriateness in a deeply personal expression, such as singing in the church choir. For others, it is an engaging discussion group with no particular religious overtone. Still others meditate and explore spiritual feelings more internally. The opportunities are vast, and each CAM program can offer some of these things, but must also keep a complete list of possible offerings in the local area. Look for the easily overlooked: nature groups or animal rescue groups can deliver the connections or "union" with the rest of the world that offer opportunities for spiritual enlightenment.

Client/Patient Health Plan

Client Name & Identifying No. ___Joe Smith___ Date of clinic team meeting: __02/02/02__
Practitioners: _Robert Roush, Primary; Jane Doe, Yoga; Rose Nilon, Reflexology; Bob Cooke,_
Chiropractor; Elaine Fob, Psychologist _____ Buddy: _Ted Jones_

Risk Factors and Plan
Causes
Internal
      Physiological—
      Enduring auto accident injuries

      Plan to reduce symptoms:
      Referral to chiropractor
      Yoga classes, reflexology

      Psychological—
      Coping skills learned/not learned in childhood

      Plan to reduce symptoms:
      Guided and personal meditation

External
      Physiological—
      Enduring auto accident injuries

      Plan to reduce symptoms:
      Concentrate on any enduring injuries from the auto accident and make a plan for
      final healing, and include such approaches as massage, chiropractic, reflexology,
      and the nutritional support for such healing to take place (e.g., a complete
      multimineral supplement with trace minerals, due to minerals' roles in building
      bones and muscle contraction).

      Psychosocial—
      Patient's attitude toward the perceptions of others and their feelings about his
      sexuality and mannerisms

      Plan to reduce symptoms:
      Minor psychotherapy and cognitive therapy, including hypnosis and role-play
      Engage in activities that make patient feel good about himself.

FIGURE 4.3. A sample health plan for a client with anal fissure (ICD9 565.0).
The plan is based on an actual health consultee of the author altered to protect
confidentiality.

Client/Patient Health Plan
Page 2

Risk Factors and Plan
Triggers (Primary Prevention Issues)
Internal
      Physiological—
      Food sensitivity

      Plan to reduce symptoms:

        1. Take note of foods that may cause a burning or itching in the rectum upon passing.

        2. Keep the area bathed and clean of waste.

      Psychospiritual—
      Life stresses are causing a "holding back" or an indecision of what to do (a spasm). The blood and the tearing might lead to the question: "What about my life is making me so angry, but feel so helpless?"

      Plan to reduce symptoms:
      Affirmation neurolinguistic programming: "I am the decision maker in control of my life, able to decide what I do, who I do it with, and when I do it!"

External
      Physiological—
      Spasm of the sphincter, causing a tear in the anal wall

      Plan to reduce symptoms:

        1. Become aware of the sphincter muscle and its tensions and contractions.

        2. Consciously relax the sphincter muscle several times per day. Have check-in sessions.

      Psychological—
      Poor work relationships, unfulfilled personal potential

      Plan to reduce symptoms:
      Making life changes, such as changing a job or a partner.
      Decide on what would self-actualize the patient.

Recommendations to Health Care Consumers

The initial recommendations can flow from the discipline of the practitioner performing the initial assessment, but a thorough understanding of the disciplines of other practitioners at the clinic should also be used. A single fee can be charged for a thorough course of treatment regardless of which modalities are used. This may assist in drawing attention away from making appointments with separate practitioners at a spiraling cost, the upper limit of which is unknown to the patient. Of course, variations in costs will arise—a course that requires eight weeks of tai chi would cost more than a course without.

Obtain permission from the client to discuss his or her needs in confidence with other practitioners during a weekly practitioner meeting. The intake practitioners should present their cases, along with their initial recommendations, and with their thoughts on referrals to other modalities, but should remain open to the suggestions of other members of the team who may have an intervention within their discipline that is unknown to the others. For example, massage therapists may feel they can be of use in the treatment of a patient with Parkinson's disease, even though it may not have been one of the original ideas of the intake practitioner. At this time, schedule a six-month follow-up appointment with the client.

At the initial intake it should be recommended to clients to keep a pad of paper and a pencil by their bedside in order to record any dreams they may have for a six-month period. Dreams are useful in diagnosis of disease (Dossey, 1999) and for improving interpersonal relationships.

Referrals and Second Recommendations

After an initial intake, the practitioner who performed this assessment may feel it is inappropriate to continue as the primary practitioner and may refer the client to another practitioner more suited to his or her needs. If a trusting relationship is being established between the two and the patient is reluctant to change the relationship, it is possible for a practitioner to continue in the role as primary contact and communicator, even if the health plan recommendations are primarily the ideas of another practitioner. If this is the case, it is still a good idea to introduce the client to the practitioner providing the most recommendations. This direct exchange between a health care practitioner and a patient is preferable, otherwise the relationship becomes similar to the concept of looking up concerns in a book and doing what the book suggests. A large part of care is the human element, and the intent for wellness that two people can formulate together.

Other initial referrals may be made immediately. For example, a homeopath performing an intake may feel that a referral to a chiropractor is required for back pain.

Once the patient receives the initial recommendations, she or he is asked to sign a release, giving permission to discuss the case with a team of practitioners (usually in daily meetings at busy clinics). It is a recommendation of this book to formulate secondary recommendations and referrals from this initial meeting within seventy-two hours. In other words, the patient should be notified, when the initial recommendations are made by the primary provider, regarding when a second set of recommendations will be made after a thorough review and discussion of the intake. A second appointment may be scheduled, or secondary recommendations may be faxed, mailed, e-mailed, or relayed by phoned. Such a clinic feature will limit practitioner income, as review time will be needed where paying appointments could be scheduled. Some cases will not require a lot of review time; others, especially those for chronic health conditions, will need ample review. The author still believes that a significant living can be earned with this approach. After all, psychology professionals who spend a full hour with clients each week can earn a significant living.

Buddy/Mentor Support System

This particular concept will be foreign to most health care practitioners who have not had some connection to the social service world. The concept of a buddy or mentor has been used successfully for decades in programs such as Alcoholics Anonymous, Big Brothers and Big Sisters of America, RSVP (Retired and Senior Volunteer Program) elderly visitation, and COMPEER, a program of friends for those suffering with mental health problems. Cancer and AIDS support groups have also used mentoring with much success. A buddy or mentor is especially useful for clients who cannot be referred to a support group for their particular conditions.

Clinics that are nonprofit and even for-profit clinics may recruit volunteers from the community, but can especially draw from current and former clients who would benefit from sharing experiences with someone who is experiencing similar difficulties with their health. The health assessment in Appendix D can be used to help match people if it is set up in a database. This way people with similarities as well as people with differences could be considered; balancing strengths could be made into matches for a buddy/mentor program. Buddies are individuals in a similar health situation, and mentors are these who have had some success in overcoming or living with their condition.

Training for a buddy/mentor program can last anywhere from a basic four-hour training to thirty-six or more hours. Buddies/mentors usually report to a volunteer coordinator. In this setting they may gain assistance, if necessary, from the primary practitioner for the client/friend. Sometimes support groups for buddies/mentors may be used to augment this role. Such programs are beyond the scope of this work and can have detailed instructor's manuals and guides running hundreds of pages. Materials from many programs can be adapted and replicated. When doing this, it is recommended to start with materials from disease-specific organizations, such as those for cancer or AIDS, because they deal with training for support in continuing health regimens and training to cope with side effects of ncessary medications. This work does not endorse one program over another, but in training for friendliness and how to be a supportive friend, the materials from COMPEER are recommended.

Following is a list of recommendations for buddies and mentors to get a program started right away. Four hours of training (one four-hour session on a Saturday, or two two-hour evening sessions) is recommended to start.

- Do not directly discuss or "dwell on" illness for any length of time.
- Do discuss treatments and treatment options, and how they are going.
- Do not suggest changing or altering treatments without discussing the ideas with your volunteer coordinator.
- Do engage in quality time not related to illness, but related to common interests, such as movies, walking, sports, hobbies.
- Do listen when times are tough.
- Do report lapses in the health plan or worsened health to the health care practitioner.
- Do engage in health plan activities, such as meditation class or even sinus cleaning together.

- Do not push too hard or let your friend be self-punishing or scolding when health plan goals are not reached.
- Do discuss modifying unrealistic health goals and write down ideas to share with the health care practitioner.
- Do share health care plans with buddies, and support each other in personal and plan goals.
- Do feel free to socialize and engage in group activities with the client/friend.
- Do not give gifts, purchase or pay for dining activities, or pay for health care or any other items for your friend.
- Do cook and share your favorite healthy dishes with your friend.
- Do attempt to share and explore spiritual goals with your friend.
- Do not become romantically involved with your friend, or try to solve familial or other problems.
- Do discuss problems but do so with a plan of how to approach them, relying on the health care practitioner for assistance.

Group Work and Classes

Group work and/or classes are recommended for all participants. These classes or group work should focus on the self-awareness and help the patient focus in the present as the decision maker in his or her own health care. Yoga, tai chi, chi gung, and group therapy support sessions can help to accomplish this. CAM programs can use this opportunity to formalize the relationship between music/art and therapy by teaching patients how to use the arts to induce relaxation or to work through difficult emotions. Some patients will want to register for disease-specific support groups in their community, taking care to select one that does not dwell too much on negative aspects of the disease. It is the author's experience that support groups for chronic and especially fatal diseases can become gripe sessions, which expend energy on the repeated expression of frustration and anger. This does not allow for mental, emotional, and spiritual healing and will certainly slow physical improvement as well.

Many community colleges and schools associated with massage now offer CAM-type courses. If your practitioner has recommended homeopathy, it is an excellent idea for the client who is unfamiliar with homeopathy to take a course in it.

All these activities are aimed at improving the knowledge and self-awareness of the patient in order for them to take charge of his or her health.

Six-Month Check-In

All patients should be scheduled for a six-month check-in. These are health and lifestyle improvement plans, and not diagnoses aimed at curing illness. The program works with physicians whose aim may be to treat the illness directly, and both a health plan and the physician treatment will do well to schedule a review halfway through a year-long plan.

The practitioner and client should review the dream journal kept by the client. At this time an analysis should be made of any dream imagery that might point to underlying psychological or physiological causes to disease. The client should be the one interpreting the meanings under the guidance of the practitioner. The practitioner should be wary of any denial involving very clear imagery. For example, the client might write: "I dreamed my heart was clogged and could not beat." Then quickly follow up with, "But I'm sure my heart is fine." If heart disease is even remotely suspected, the client should follow up with a cardiologist. From the psychological standpoint, the client may wish to explore any impediments he or she may have in expressing love.

Some of the practices in the plan are meant to be permanent, but others may be temporary. What were the results of the plan and how should it be readjusted, so that the original goals can be achieved in another six months? At this time, it might also be necessary to reevaluate some goals. At any rate, a new plan is written at this time. If no changes are necessary and everything is perfectly in line, then it is recommended to increase or make some goals *more* ambitious. This is the time to make the changes.

One-Year Check-In

At the end of one year, the client receives a final statement and recommendation for continuing health care practices. At this time any remaining issues may be clarified and answered. Achievements can be chronicled. The CAM clinic at this point has the option of issuing a certificate of completion for the healthy lifestyle goals that were achieved. One full year of a program which contains built-in follow-up and support networks that encourage true behavioral change is more likely to have a higher success rate than quick visitation for point-of-demand health considerations. Even one long single appointment with a conscientious health care practitioner is not as likely to be as successful as such a program.

Pricing

It is not likely that this advice on pricing will help to change the wildly divergent approach to charging clients for services in CAM. This clinic design does offer the opportunity to charge one price for a full year course of sessions, including one set of classes and some visits to other practitioners. One possible approach would be similar to a health club membership, where a monthly fee is charged, and certain services are rendered for that fee. Although this could not include unlimited service, it could include one monthly visit to any practitioner deemed necessary at that time. Such a set of charges for the complete course of treatment might break down this way:

1. Initial assessment and recommendations	$50.00
2. Follow-up recommendations	$40.00
3. Eight-week class, then monthly thereafter (a total of 18 sessions)	$180.00
4. Monthly practitioner visit (i.e., Reiki, massage, etc.)	$480.00
5. Six-month follow-up	$50.00
6. End evaluation	$50.00
TOTAL	$850.00

This averages about $71 per month, very reasonable in comparison to a health club. Of course, any prices may be set for these individual services depending on the location and the amount that it is necessary to charge. Perhaps a highly reputable program in an expensive city might cost $225 per month. The point is that people can pay a monthly fee and receive a large range of services on a regular basis throughout the year. Such plans might even be marketable and popular to give as gifts, just as health club memberships are. In other words, a good health clinic structure based solely on the health considerations of an individual can make good marketing sense as well.

One future for such a program—when data can be gathered to support the hypothesis of improved health and reduced future health care costs for its participants—is to offer such a program as part of a health insurance premium that includes all emergency and other care.

Third-Party Reimbursement/Insurance

CAM practitioners have cited the opportunity (or inopportunity, as it were) to charge insurance carriers and Medicaid/Medicare assistance as one of its main obstacles to growth (see Chapter 2). If the system described is adopted and supervised by a licensed professional, the argument to health insurance companies is strengthened because each relative cause and triggering factor is assessed and documented. All the physical interventions can become allowable under the descriptions of physical therapy that are given by the insurance providers. Even when unlicensed practitioners are functioning as the primary provider, a clinic with a licensed medical director who takes responsibility for supervising individuals can make complete plans that are reimbursable by insurance carriers. A complete list of International Classification of Disease, Ninth Edition (ICD-9) diagnostic codes and allowable procedural codes should be obtained from the insurance providers. Insurance billing is a complex affair beyond the scope of this work, however commercial software and provider-created databases can house this information in relation to each insurance provider and can be checked to be sure billing and procedures match the insurer's requirements.

For practitioners not authorized to bill insurance under current laws and insurer regulations, this work would, most likely, require the establishment of licensing or standardized certification for the modalities (as described in Chapter 3), and then the convincing of insurance companies to allow billing from these practitioners. Only two things can cause such a revolution: (1) proof that such modalities and such systems reduce costs for insurance carriers in the long run and (2) consumer demand for insurance that allows such coverage, with consumers refusing insurance that does not offer such coverage. Both achievements will be difficult to bring about and will require massive organization from individual groups calling for the licensing or standardized certification of modalities, and from consumer groups and businesses purchasing health insurance. The involvement of the government in such issues, especially a single authority such as the NIH's NCCAM will speed such achievements.

CONCLUSION

This chapter introduced the concept of applying the five domains of CAM to a thorough health assessment and creation of a healthy lifestyle plan. The exhaustive nature of the assessment and written plan is dependent on an understanding of illness that differentiates between illness causes and triggers and further differentiates between internal and external influences, broken down into physiological, psychological, social, and spiritual realms within these internal and external influences. Regular clinic visits with appropriate CAM modalities, support groups, classes, and a buddy/mentor support system will ensure the achievement of an individual's health goals over the period of one year.

Chapter 5

Needed Research, Suggestions, and Speculations

FURTHER RESEARCH

Doing a large research project and making suggestions for overall improvement in a field invariably leads to more questions and the need for further research.

The most unwieldy thing about CAM, even when broken down into five fairly reasonable and understandable domains, is its vast, almost absurd, disparity. How can treatments for one person and essentially one illness be inclusive of different treatment such as prescription drugs, surgery, meditation, biofeedback, music therapy, Reiki, and prayer? For some the answer is obvious; yet others will consider such a regimen to contain good treatment options but also options which may lead to no harm but are ineffective. Still others will find this regimen to contain highly harmful or misleading treatments— either from the perspective of the pure holism camp or the pure conventional medical science camp.

It is this author's contention that most practitioners are moderate in their beliefs, and that it is time for these moderates to sweep into the middle, engulf the extremes on either end, and give patients the vast, rich repertoire that is available right now, based on the accumulated knowledge of thousands of years and many cultures. This book is meant to be a tool to access such powerful options, if not the vehicle to initiate such a revolution.

More study needs to be done to determine exactly how certain modalities *complement* and *integrate* with one another. How can a dose of muscle relaxant be combined with massage to ease pain and make joints and lumbar return to their desired position? How can herbs and expressive arts therapy combine to alleviate depression? The CAM combinations are endless. The potential for relief is monumental.

This book's health assessment tool and model for illness leading to a health plan needs to be implemented and studied on a wider scale, using clinical experience to refine and improve the system. It can be done in a conscientious way, but it will take the participation of many clinics and many patients. The open-minded and willing experimental approach of CAM practitioners is not the only required ingredient. Patients can no longer be considered patients and must instead be clients—clients who actively participate in their own health choices. This process of how clients participate and why they will make certain health choices must also be studied. Can we get a handle on the personal processes that will lead to solving complicated health problems, with different causes, triggers, and roots within a client's personal makeup? The clients are the city where such cures take place, and the practitioners are merely the mapmakers. Imagine, if you will, a world in which health discoveries are named after the *person who overcame the problem* rather than the practitioner who supposedly suggested the cure. Researchers and health care providers are those who will document and formalize the procedures.

DECREASING LITIGATION

Increased medical litigation is no surprise to anyone in any state in the United States. Pennsylvania, for example, is an increasingly difficult state in which to pay for medical malpractice insurance (La Torre, 2001). This has caused physicians to leave the state and look elsewhere to practice. Recent attention has been brought to this because of the decision of the Philadelphia court system to catch up on its backlog of malpractice suits. It was noted in May 2001 that premiums for insurance have risen another 25 percent beyond the already $60,000 or more per year. Some say that medical errors still cause more deaths than either AIDS or motor vehicle accidents, and that physicians are failing to discipline their own, in addition to failing to come up with ways to decrease such statistics.

From 1991 to 1999, Pennsylvania was second only to New York State in the amount patients collected from malpractice settlements. Public distrust of the medical profession includes such ugliness as the ruling in October 2001 that TAP Pharmaceutical pay $840 million to settle allegations that the company hiked its prices and bribed doctors to prescribe Lupron Depot, a prostate cancer drug. Such racketeering must stop. Laws requiring preventive health care, and a system that tries milder forms of intervention before powerful and dangerous drugs, should be instituted. The clinic structure recommended in this book is designed for instituting such a system.

Decreasing litigation is a goal of physicians, hospitals, and insurance companies alike. The idea of a patient becoming a client and discarding the idea of "waiting patiently while the doctor does stuff" is the start to decreasing litigation. As mentioned, the patient has the attitude that, "I'm your partner in my care until something goes wrong. Then you're responsible." This is the perfect litigious attitude. Moving the patient away from this attitude toward that of a responsible client or consumer is not a single-step or one-sided process. Consumers in the United States love to sue businesses as well, but not as often, and not for quite as much money. When life and death issues are involved, little can prevent citizens from taking advantage of the law in order to compensate for losses. Indeed, when true gross negligence and incompetence does cause harm, it helps no one to simply make lawsuits more difficult to pursue.

One of the factors in the industry that is important to note is the extreme cost of health care. It is shocking and can devastate an entire family's lives, especially if third-party insurance coverage is either nonexistent or insufficient. Partially effective care might seem reasonable at the price of several hundred or even several thousand dollars, but such care at tens of thousands or hundreds of thousands of dollars can claim every asset and can throw the litigation switch very quickly. Little to nothing has been done to check the outrageous, spiraling costs of health care. No other industry performs services for customers without divulging the cost or details of the services, then simply bills for these services *at any cost* and expects to be paid, even if the services did not work. This single factor, if not dealt with, will mean that the current litigation crisis will go on and on, ad nauseam.

The following is a list of suggestions for both consumers and health care professionals to ease and build relations at a time of crisis in the health care industry.

- Assume the clients and/or family members are capable of understanding their health, reviewing their options, and making decisions with the information that you provide for them and that you develop together.

- Establish a rapport with your client by discussing all the details and costs of options frankly, reminding the client that you are there to help facilitate a healing, which, if possible, will come from within him or her.
- Never perform a procedure without first explaining it to the client and/or family members.
- Provide a mechanism to assist clients in paying for the care you feel they may truly need (even if this just means consultation on all their payment options). Be frank about the risks of refusing or not engaging in care simply because it may seem too expensive.
- Be frank about successes and limitations known in the field and with the procedures recommended.
- Be frank about your own weaknesses. Consult with others for the benefit of your client.
- When things go wrong, speculate with the client on what might be the problem.
- Admit mistakes. That is correct. This goes against any legal advice you may have heard in the past, but part of building a relationship with your client means being a fallible fellow human being.
- Strive to provide more complete, comprehensive care at a reasonable price (see the health assessment and health plan approach in Chapter 4).
- After establishing a relationship, elect to voluntarily disclose your malpractice history. Explain to clients why you may have won or lost, and especially why you think you were sued in the first place.

Political activity and tort reform have a chance of survival if they do not seek to cap either attorney's fees or awards for malpractice. This makes it rather obvious that money is the issue—as in saving it for insurance companies and physicians. The public and the courts are not interested in this. Instead, reform legislation should list reasonable complications of various medical procedures, and require patients to be informed of the possible complications that are beyond the control of the physicians. There should be limits to what patients can sue for (if anything) when their own behavior has put them in a dangerous or life-threatening situation. Emergency-room doctors should have some "Good Samaritan" protection, and there should be solid evidence of gross negligence before such cases can proceed to court.

On the other side of the coin, doctors should make checklists for medical errors that can cause harm, and check them once and then twice in the execution of their duties. The statistics on the types of harm the courts compensate for is available from insurance companies who provide malpractice coverage. There is no question that a reality check is essential: this includes a reasonable price structure for medical care and a change in the perception that doctors are deeppocketed beings who should be infallible.

Research surrounds any given concept with abundant information from which judgments can be made about how something actually operates in the world. Research can be counted for or against a concept much as a court weighs evidence for and against a defendant in order to make a decision about what really happened.

For example, one study reported in the *New England Journal of Medicine* cast some doubt on the nature of the placebo effect (Hrobjartsson and Gotzsche, 2001), something that has been long established in the scientific community as having a strong bearing on the outcomes of health and efficacy trials. The study reported that, "As compared with no treatment, placebo had no significant effect on binary outcomes, regardless of whether these outcomes were subjective or objective. For the trials with continuous outcomes, placebo had a beneficial effect, but the effect decreased with increasing sample size, indicating a possible bias related to the effects of small trials" (p. 1594). In addition, "In 27 trials involving the treatment of pain, placebo had a beneficial effect, as indicated by a reduction in the intensity of pain" (p. 1594). The study concluded that, "We found little evidence in general that placebos had powerful clinical effects. Although placebos had no significant effects on objective or binary outcomes, they had possible small benefits in studies with continuous subjective outcomes and for the treatment of pain. Outside the setting of clinical trials, there is no justification for the use of placebos" (p. 1594). But who on earth applies the use of placebos *extensively* in clinical *practice?* It is well known that the same diminishing quality exists for extensive research in larger sample sizes for substances that are proven relatively effective.

This study is mentioned here in order to compare it to a news arti-cle about it released by the Associated Press, by author Linda A. Johnson. The article appeared in May 2001 (Johnson, 2001) and stated that researchers "found little or no placebo effect in dozens of trials" (p. A9) and was titled "Study Scoffs at Placebo Effect." This headline was apparently added by the source *(The Morning Call)* as it is listed in the online Lexis-Nexis database of new stories as "Study Questions Placebo Response." The article went on to quote John C. Bailar III, a retired professor of health studies at the University of Chicago, as stating, "The shoe is on the other foot now. The people who claim there are placebo effects are going to have to show it" (p. A9). The entire article was written from the angle that the concept of placebo effect had just been eradicated from science. The average person would find it difficult to get any other impression from this ar-ticle, but clearly, when compared to the *New England Journal of Medicine* article, the conclusions quoted here are far from the truth. The actual study found a quite powerful effect for pain relief. The strongest statement against the *existence* of a placebo effect was, "For the trials with continuous outcomes, placebo had a beneficial effect, but the effect decreased with increasing sample size" (p. 1594). This is very different from scoffing at placebo effect.

The message? Both the public and health care practitioners should be very wary of press reports about health topics. Journalists look for "slants," often at the expense of equally weighing information in a study—something that is crucial if there is to be a true understanding of the possibilities. Sometimes they just get the slant wrong or skew it enough so that the information given becomes meaningless. Yet peo-ple make decisions and take action on health matters based on what is reported in the press daily. What then is a reasonable approach for the public, health care practitioners, and the press in educating the con-sumer about CAM or really *any* health product or service?

CONSUMER EDUCATION

Health care practitioners and consumers can take steps to be sure that they are getting the best information possible about health care options. One approach consumers should have is to ally themselves with health programs and their family physicians in order to discuss issues and ideas as they are presented in the press. The CAM clinic approach described here is one possible way to find practitioners willing to discuss popular slants on health care.

Once an issue takes hold in the press—that is to say, that the public seems to be looking for more information on the subject—the press, true to its craft, will increase research on the subject, asking more experts for their opinion and uncovering medical research and government reports. At its best, the media has shed light on health subjects and has truly changed both public and professional opinion. One such example has been its alliance with community grassroots groups to change perceptions and behavior in regard to heart disease. Exercise, cholesterol levels, stress levels, and diet have been covered, reiterated, and covered again. In part, this exposure has led to a consumer consciousness and public awareness of CAM that has grown along with the media reports. In this instance, the popularity of CAM has been intertwined with public interest health matters and consumer desire for relatively low-cost health solutions.

The approach for conventional medicine toward CAM has been the opposite in many respects, drawing on an authoritarian role that it still relies on, even when all the evidence is pointing away from their stance. A good indicator that conventional medicine has run out of arguments against CAM is often quoted as something to the effect, "No studies about this have been published in reputable medical journals . . ." which really just arrogantly states, "We'll decide what's significant in medicine: We own the journals and control their content. *We'll* let *you* know when something significant in medicine occurs." These journals withhold information from the public, and what they do publish is often in unfamiliar terms. Licensing still ensures that only people from this camp of scientific medicine be consulted to diagnose and treat illness, keeping control over their corner on the market. Yet the market is out of control and patients are self-treating and self-referring at a level that is at least equal with conventional medical care. If medicine and hospitals were to remove treatment for problems caused by their own treatments, it could be argued that the public utilizes *more* self-treatment than conventional medical treatment and, as discussed, the heads of families (usually female) are in charge of this care.

Therefore, we now know to *whom* we are marketing: caretakers in families—and these caretakers are more open to CAM than ever before. Yet confusion exists over CAM and what its potential is. Drug companies are aggressively marketing products to the public in repeated advertisements because they are now aware that direct consumer marketing in health is the way to go. However, a balance is necessary because visiting your physician merely to get a prescription you saw advertised on television is the tail wagging the dog. If we were to have a law requiring milder, natural remedies as intervention *before* these medications, it would force the same requirement for safety and efficacy that is now required for drugs to be applied to herbs and nutritional products as well. This does not mean they have to be regulated the same way as prescription drugs in their sales, but that they must meet some type of standard for quality and efficacy. This would be a solution that extremes on both sides would be against; the nutraceutical and herbal industries would be against the standards and the AMA would be against the requirement for these remedies as a front line of defense. In the United States, the most powerful lobby often prevails—as opposed to the best line of thinking. This reduces the argument about health to one between two powerful industries and they are both the industries that make pill-form, gastrointestinal tract options in health care.

The answers and options for educating the public about CAM and how it is about more than pills lies in the same solution that eventually drew treatment for heart disease out of the realm of medicine and into the realm of prevention. A strong national organization must gain a hold, much as the American Heart Association did in the 1920s (but especially as its post-WWII reorganization), and begin to systematically perform research and educate the public. The government's efforts with NCCAM is only the beginning. The public must become aroused enough to start an organization at the grassroots level. To clarify, this organization would *not* be a professional organization per se but would consist of public and professional members.

Such organizations rally around a central health cause to convey a powerful message, and this cause usually involves death or severe impairment for a single disease or group of diseases. CAM can rally around the loss of and lack of quality of life and emphasize longevity. It is therefore recommended that one of the organizations concerned with longevity devote itself to sorting out how CAM and traditional medicine integrate to provide the most complete health care ever known.

Individual CAM providers can ally themselves with longevity efforts in their own locale and seek to find a powerful national voice to join, speaking out about prevention and longevity in all of health care. They can rally to write letters to the editor about important health matters in their community, and begin to join speakers' bureaus that address small community groups. Local volunteer agencies and the United Way, as well as disease-specific organizations have these speakers' bureaus. This is volunteer work to be sure, but it is crucial if education is to lay a foundation in the roots of the community.

Advertising is a last and expensive resort. Instead, local colleges and universities should offer courses and discussion forums, and foster an intellectual discourse on CAM. Finally, universities should establish departments that offer training in the CAM modalities in order to bring about the earliest community standards in training for CAM.

The puzzle pieces will either fall into place as more legislation occurs and as the battle between camps heats up—or the heat of the extremes will fizzle from pressure from the middle. Let us hope it is the latter.

FINAL SPECULATIONS

One wonders if new scientific advances will once again negate CAM as effective, the way the discovery of antibiotics and scientific medicine supposedly squelched it before. Time revealed that the forthcoming breakthrough cures that were supposed to follow on the heels of antibiotics never appeared: But what of something such as genetic research, which seems to hold so much promise? Even if such research proves that the condition of our mind and even our approach to spiritualism can be reconciled through the adjustment of our genetic code (which is doubtful), it still cannot scale the wall of the old argument against nature versus nurture. In other words, finding all the solutions within the realm of genetics would mean that genetics rules over our health 100 percent. Instead, our personal choices and prevention activities in all likelihood will still remain equally important; despite the use of genetics to strengthen our bodies, we are likely to still die if we jump from airplanes without parachutes. Preventive and thorough health assessment based on multiple traditions will likely be needed even more as we enter into the worlds of more brave science.

EPILOGUE

Finally, gaining greater health is about hope for the future. Yet the future remains inextricably linked to the past, and many people with severe health problems will say that they cannot turn back the hands of time—to prevent an accident from happening, to stop themselves from being infected with a deadly disease, or to halt the development of cancer or heart disease. However, isn't genetic research about changing the past? Doesn't our new ability to manipulate genes allow us to now change things we never thought we could? This brings up the idea that if we could somehow alter the past, we could make things better for ourselves.

Here is a dream the author had:

> In a dream, I was traveling into the past with my present person (body) sliding or falling, suspended in a tube with levels or floors. Each floor I passed was perhaps a year or annual cycle.
>
> Superimposed on the dream was the image of a formula, or markings depicting what had occurred, such as:
>
> K y l l m p t 23
>
> Then, a second formula was superimposed directly on top of the old formula, which showed how I had influenced the past:
>
> KyLLMpT23
>
> Uppercased letters indicated a change to the past.
>
> I awoke and reviewed the dream in my mind, concluding it meant the past could be influenced via the present. I wondered why I would dream such a thing, and if I were mad.

Although my conclusion seems outrageous on the surface, some other mysteries seem improbable as well. It is a great mystery of physics that light (photons) behaves as particles or a wave, depending on what the physicist is looking for. One well-known physics experiment is performed by firing laser photons randomly through two different slats at a semipenetrating mirror. Half the light goes through and half is reflected. Because of the different distances traveled, an interference pattern occurs that is detected by an instrument set up to do so. This pattern is much like the ripples that occur when one throws a stone into water followed closely by a second stone of similar size: the two sets of waves that the stones make collide and "cancel" each other out. The pattern remains when only one photon is sent at a time. When the mirror is removed the interference pattern disappears. In addition, when the device attempts to detect which of the two slits a particle travels through, the interference pattern also disappears.

When the device detects at the last moment whether it will measure the passing of a particle (so fast that the light must have already passed the semipenetrating mirror, and part of the light wave is already under way in the other direction) the interference pattern also disappears. This means that the light wave that was already under way in the other direction must have been stopped in its tracks somehow. In other words, the past is changed by a decision in the present.

Examples of this phenomenon are not limited to photons. If the photon experiment is difficult to follow or you are skeptical of the conclusion that the past can be changed from the present, consider the research done by the Princeton Engineering Anomalies Research (PEAR) Facility. Literally millions of trials have occurred in almost thirty years. In the 1970s a project was started to see what the effect of *intention* was on an electronic device. Most often studied is the effect of intention on a device known as a random events generator (REG). The REG is switched on and records an endless stream of randomly generated pluses and minuses. It is set to generate an equal number over a fairly short period of time. It also records the precise time the events (the recording of a plus or minus) were generated. The experiment may last for days. A person who tries to influence the experiment will try to create more pluses or more minuses. Over time it was concluded that not only was there a statistically significant ability to influence the results, but that results recorded in the past were influenced by intentions at some future point (Dossey, 1999). One important feature is that the results, though real, were limited—the stream of pluses and minuses is never changed entirely to one character or the other.

Thus the author's dream appears accurate: there are minor but significant changes to the past; the dream described a specific way in which the past might be changed but that there might be a limit: any change would still be based on what had previously occurred.

But how do these experiments indicate we can really change our *own* past, and how does this give us hope for the future? Recently, the author came across writings that, it is claimed, were channeled from other beings through Kieran Rowser (Rowser, 1999). These writings are concerned with the idea that people have the power to change the past. They note that if

> suffering becomes eliminated from the vocabulary, from the conceptual mind, then that also eliminates it in the future . . . We're saying [this is] literally seeing things in a different light . . . [but] we are not only talking about viewing things in a different way, but also truly, some of the really jagged stuff, shall we say, just never happened.

This solution seems to be almost overly simple for such a baffling physical and metaphysical phenomenon. It is saying that the key to changing the past is the *attitude* of the *present:* once the *meaning* of what has happened changes in the present (perhaps to a more positive and enlightened understanding) the past thus changes to meet our understanding in the present. This means we can influence our health through such enlightened viewing. As the director of an AIDS center in Bethlehem, Pennsylvania, the author has had countless opportunities to hear AIDS patients make such declarations as, "Getting AIDS was the best thing that ever happened to me," and "I was never well until I got AIDS." These patients, in the revelation brought on by their illness, found that the past experience of acquiring such a disease was not as horrific or "jagged" as they had previously thought. In fact, it was *good*.

May we all harness such power in our lives!

Appendix A

Patient Raw Data

N = 438. Wherever percentages add to more than 100 percent, multiple answers were given.

Gender	Number	Percent
Female	369	84.25
Male	46	10.50
No answer	23	5.25

Education		
Some high school	111	25.34
High school grad/GED	143	32.65
Some college	91	20.78
Two-year degree	27	6.16
Four-year degree	31	7.08
Graduate school	23	5.25
No answer	12	2.74

Age		
18-29	160	36.53
30-40	120	27.40
41-50	46	10.50
51-60	23	5.25
61-70	13	2.97
71+	32	7.31
No answer	44	10.05

Household Income		
Under $10,000	119	27.17
$10,000-20,000	99	22.60
$20,000-30,000	57	13.01
$30,000-40,000	27	6.16

	Number	Percent
$40,000-50,000	14	3.20
$50,000-70,000	30	6.85
$70,000-90,000	18	4.11
$90,000+	12	2.74
No answer	62	14.16

Number in Household

	Number	Percent
4	114	26.03
3	103	23.52
2	79	18.04
1	51	11.64
5	43	9.82
6	17	3.88
7	11	2.51
8	6	1.37
9	2	0.46
No answer	12	2.74

Do you have any of the following conditions?
(n = 437)

	Number	Percent
Overweight	140	32.04
Headaches	90	20.59
Anxiety	93	21.28
Allergy	78	17.85
Fatigue	57	13.04
High blood pressure	73	16.70
Sinusitis	42	9.61
Arthritis	45	10.30
Asthma	49	11.21
Interpersonal relations	32	7.32
High cholesterol	37	8.47
Heart	34	7.78
Irritable bowel	21	4.81
Diabetes	28	6.41
Attention deficit	9	2.06
Osteoporosis	9	2.06
Cancer	4	0.92
Fibromyalgia	2	0.46

	Number	Percent

Do you take prescription and/or over-the-counter (OTC) medication? (n = 438)

Yes	227	51.83
No	190	43.38
No answer	21	4.79

If so, how many different prescriptions do you take a day? (n = 210)

1 per day	86	40.95
2-3 per day	74	35.24
3-5 per day	30	14.29
5+ per day	20	9.52

Do you take any vitamin/mineral supplements? (n = 220)

Yes		50.34
Multivitamins	151	68.64
Vitamin E	32	14.55
Vitamin C	29	13.18
Calcium	21	9.55
Vitamin Bs	17	7.73
Centrum	16	7.27
Iron supplement	6	2.73
Folic acid	4	1.82
Glucosamine sulfate	4	1.82
Garlic	3	1.36
Magnesium malate	3	1.36
Vitamin A	3	1.36
CoQ10	2	0.91
Antioxidant	1	0.45
Chitosan	1	0.45
Chondroitin	1	0.45
Chromium picolinate	1	0.45
Fish oil	1	0.45
Grape seed	1	0.45
K-Dur	1	0.45
Lactobacillus	1	0.45

	Number	**Percent**
Lecithin	1	0.45
Melatonin	1	0.45
Selenium	1	0.45
Soy protein	1	0.45
Vitamin D	1	0.45
Zinc	1	0.45

Do you take any herbal supplements? Please list.
(n = 40)

Yes		11.67
St. John's wort	5	12.50
Echinacea	4	10.00
Ginseng	3	7.50
Black cohosh	2	5.00
Chamomile	2	5.00
Feverfew	2	5.00
Garlic	2	5.00
Ginkgo biloba	2	5.00
Juniper berry	2	5.00
Black walnut	1	2.50
Butcher's broom	1	2.50
Chromium	1	2.50
Citrimax	1	2.50
Dongerai	1	2.50
Flax seed	1	2.50
Fo-ti	1	2.50
Ling	1	2.50
Glucosamine sulfate	1	2.50
Green tea	1	2.50
Herbal athlete's formula	1	2.50
Kava	1	2.50
Milk thistle	1	2.50
Peppermint	1	2.50
Primrose oil	1	2.50
Thermagenics	1	2.50
Thermalift	1	2.50
Uva ursi	1	2.50
Yellow dock	1	2.50

	Number	Percent
Where do you purchase these supplements? **(n = 225)**		
Pharmacy	89	39.56
Grocery store	86	38.22
No answer	49	21.78
Health food store	30	13.33
Mail order	22	9.78

	Number	Percent
Do you use any of the following services? **(n = 438)**		
Yes	152	34.70

	Number	**Percent of Sample (n = 152)**	**Percent of Total (n = 438)**
Prayer	99	65.13	22.60
Music	40	26.32	9.13
Chiropractic	34	22.37	7.76
Psychology	23	15.13	5.25
Nutrition	21	13.82	4.79
Pastoral counseling	17	11.18	3.88
Meditation	16	10.53	3.65
Massage	14	9.21	3.20
Aromatherapy	11	7.24	2.51
Mind/body	6	3.95	1.37
Yoga	6	3.95	1.37
Reflexology	6	3.95	1.37
Reiki	5	3.29	1.14
Homeopathy	4	2.63	0.91
Herbs	3	1.97	0.68
Acupuncture	3	1.97	0.68
Chinese	1	0.66	0.23
Ayurvedic	1	0.66	0.23
Naturopathy	0	0.00	0.00

If you use any of these methods, please circle your source of information. (n = 102)	Number	Percent
Newspaper/radio/TV	51	50.00
Family physician	38	37.25

	Number	Percent
Computer/Internet	26	25.49
Magazine	24	23.53
Health care practitioner	23	22.55
Health food store	18	17.65
Newsletter	9	8.82

What, if any, would you be interested in learning more about? (n = 438)

| | | 158 | 36.07 |

	Number	Percent of Sample (n = 158)	Percent of Total (n = 438)
Nutrition	49	31.01	11.19
Massage	39	24.68	8.90
Mind/body	37	23.42	8.45
Music	35	22.15	7.99
Yoga	28	17.72	6.39
Meditation	27	17.09	6.16
Herbs	24	15.19	5.48
Aromatherapy	24	15.19	5.48
Chiropractic	21	13.29	4.79
Prayer	20	12.66	4.57
Psychology	19	12.03	4.34
Acupuncture	19	12.03	4.34
Reflexology	18	11.39	4.11
Reiki	15	9.49	3.42
Homeopathy	15	9.49	3.42
Chinese	13	8.23	2.97
Pastoral counseling	11	6.96	2.51
Naturopathy	7	4.43	1.60
Ayurvedic	4	2.53	0.91

How would you prefer to learn about these practices? (n = 151)

	Number	Percent
Seminar by a practitioner	57	37.75
Family physician	38	25.17
Newspaper/radio/TV	37	24.50

	Number	Percent
Magazine	36	23.84
Seminar by an MD	34	22.52
Computer/Internet	33	21.85
Newsletter	22	14.57
Health food store	11	7.28

Would you be interested in attending a health fair that had information on these topics, targeting the service of those who have unresolved health issues and/or low income? (n = 438)

	Number	Percent
No	224	51.14
Yes	150	34.25
No answer	64	14.61

Appendix B

Physician Raw Data

N = 35. Responses and changes of nine or more (26 percent) may be significant.

Practitioner Type	Number	Percent
MD	11	31.43
DO	10	21.70
Specialist	3	6.52
Resident	9	19.57
No answer	2	4.35

Do you have patients with any of the following conditions?

Anxiety	31	88.57
Overweight	31	88.57
Sinusitis	31	88.57
Headaches	30	85.71
High blood pressure	30	85.71
Diabetes	30	85.71
High cholesterol	30	85.71
Fatigue	29	82.86
Heart	29	82.86
Allergy	29	82.86
Arthritis	29	82.86
Asthma	29	82.86
Irritable bowel	27	77.14
Cancer	26	74.29
Interpersonal relations	25	71.43
Attention deficit	25	71.43
Osteoporosis	25	71.43
Fibromyalgia	22	62.86

	Number	Percent
Do you prescribe medication and/or over-the-counter (OTC) medication?		
Yes	32	91.43
No	0	0.00
No answer	3	6.52
Do you prescribe any vitamin/mineral supplements? (n = 25)		
Yes		71.43
Multivitamin	20	80.00
Calcium	10	40.00
Vitamin E	8	32.00
Vitamin C	6	24.00
B-complex	3	12.00
Vitamin D	3	12.00
Folic acid	2	8.00
Antioxidants	1	4.00
Folate	1	4.00
Garlic	1	4.00
Glucosamine	1	4.00
Iron	1	4.00
MVI—allergies	1	4.00
Niacin	1	4.00
Do you prescribe any herbal supplements? (n = 9)		
Yes		25.71
St. John's wort	4	44.44
*Chondroitin	2	22.22
Gingko biloba	2	22.22
*Glucosamine	2	22.22
Goldenseal	2	22.22
"Some herbal"	2	22.22
Chamomile	1	11.11
Garlic	1	11.11
Grape seed oil	1	11.11

	Number	Percent
Melatonin	1	11.11
Passion flower	1	11.11
Saw palmetto	1	11.11

*Note: Although not technically herbal supplements, glucosamine and chondroitin were left in this section as physicians often confuse nutraceuticals (closer to vitamins) and herbs.

Where do you recommend the purchase of these supplements? (n = 22)

Pharmacy	16	72.73
Health food store	12	54.55
Grocery store	7	31.82
Mail order	3	13.64

Do you refer to any of the following services? (n = 33)

Psychology	26	74.29
Nutrition	24	68.57
Pastoral counseling	13	37.14
Prayer	10	28.57
Massage	10	28.57
Acupuncture	10	28.57
Meditation	8	22.86
Chiropractic	7	20.00
Mind/body	4	11.43
Yoga	4	11.43
Herbalist	4	11.43
Homeopathic	2	5.71
Music	1	2.86
Reflexology	1	2.86
Reiki	1	2.86
Chinese	1	2.86
Naturopathy	1	2.86
Aromatherapy	0	0.00
Ayurvedic	0	0.00

	Number	**Percent**

**If you refer to any of the above methods,
please circle your source of information (n = 28)**

	Number	Percent
Continuing education	16	57.14
Practitioner of modality	11	39.29
Computer/Internet	4	14.29
Newspaper/Radio/TV	4	14.29
Magazine	4	14.29
Health food store	2	7.14
Newsletter	1	3.57

**What, if any, would you be interested in
learning more about? (n = 28)**

	Number	Percent
Acupuncture	7	1.60
Nutrition	4	0.91
Mind/body	4	0.91
Herbs	3	0.68
Massage	2	0.46
Pastoral counseling	2	0.46
Psychology	2	0.46
Yoga	2	0.46
Reflexology	2	0.46
Naturopathy	2	0.46
Prayer	1	3.57
Music	1	0.23
Meditation	1	0.23
Homeopathic	1	0.23
Aromatherapy	1	0.23
Chiropractic	0	0.00
Reiki	0	0.00
Chinese	0	0.00
Ayurvedic	0	0.00

	Number	Percent

How would you prefer to learn about the above practices? (n = 31)

	Number	Percent
Seminar by a practitioner	20	64.52
Seminar by an MD	17	54.84
Newspaper/radio/TV	7	22.58
Computer/Internet	6	19.35
Magazine	4	12.90
Newsletter	1	3.23

Would you be interested in attending a health fair which had information on the above topics?

	Number	Percent
Yes	27	77.14
No	7	20.00
No answer	1	2.86

Appendix C

CAM Clinic Raw Data

N = 59. Statistic reminder: the relatively small sampling means that there is no statistical significance of a response or difference less than a count of nine, or 15.52 percent.

Annual gross income was not responded to by twenty-one of fifty-nine people. One respondent said, "mind your own business." Of the thirty-eight responding, income ranged from $3,000 to $600,000 dollars, with the mean being $135,000. More than half (63 percent) fell between $25,000 and $100,000.

The total number of practitioners ranged from one to twenty, with an average of four. The largest group (34 percent) was single-practitioner businesses (twenty).

Do practitioners within your CAM program collaborate on the health of a single patient/client?

Answer	Number	Percent
Yes	35	59.32
No	9	15.25
No answer	15	25.42
(mostly single practitioners)		

What is the most common format of the collaboration?

Informal communication	28	47.46
Formal meetings (structured)	7	11.86
No answer	24	40.68

What is the average hourly rate (total charged or total cost) for a practitioner at your CAM program?

The rates ranged from $15 to $360 an hour, with an average of $77.75. Clearly no standard exists for CAM modality reimbursement. Some practitioners run "traditional" practices in which "as many as possible" patients are seen in an hour. Some spent large amounts of time with patients, only painfully accepting payment. One practitioner who saw as many people as possible in an hour said that CAM practitioners often failed because "they didn't know how to run a business."

All raw data is ranked from greatest to least response.
1. Please check each heading and each modality your CAM program currently offers:

	Number	Percent
Body-Based Manipulation Therapies	40	67.80
Massage	36	61.02
Reflexology	22	37.29
Chiropractic	16	27.12
Osteopathic manipulation	5	8.47
Applied kinesiology	3	5.08
Iridology	2	3.39
Ear candling	2	3.39
Tui na	1	1.69
Biologically Based Interventions	38	64.41
Herbs	35	59.32
Diet/nutrition	35	59.32
Vitamins	32	54.24
Nutraceutical	12	20.34
Electromagnetic	12	20.34
Magnetic	8	13.56
Electrical	7	11.86
Alternative Medical Systems	37	62.71
Homeopathy	24	40.68
Chinese	21	35.59
Naturopathy	10	16.95
Ayurveda	8	13.56
Tibetan	0	0.00
Mind/Body Interventions	30	50.85
Meditation	20	33.90
Yoga	16	27.12
Chi gung	11	18.64
Biofeedback	8	13.56

	Number	Percent
Art/music therapy	8	13.56
Tai chi	7	11.86
Western psychology	4	6.78
Hypnosis	4	6.78
Aikido	1	1.69
Energy/Metaphysical Therapies	28	47.46
Prayer	6	10.17
Reiki	25	42.37
Therapeutic touch	16	27.12
Shamanism	5	8.47
Intuitive counseling	2	3.39
Chakra balancing	1	1.69
Jin shin jyutsu	1	1.69
Past-life regressions	1	1.69
Offered all 5 domains	10	16.95
Ranked by Modality:	**Number**	**Percent**
Massage	36	61.02
Herbs	35	59.32
Diet/nutrition	35	59.32
Vitamins	32	54.24
Reiki	25	42.37
Homeopathy	24	40.68
Reflexology	22	37.29
Chinese	21	35.59
Meditation	20	33.90
Chiropractic	16	27.12
Yoga	16	27.12
Therapeutic touch	16	27.12
Nutraceutical	12	20.34
Electromagnetic	12	20.34
Chi gung	11	18.64
Naturopathy	10	16.95
Magnetic	8	13.56
Ayurveda	8	13.56
Biofeedback	8	13.56
Art/music therapy	8	13.56

	Number	Percent
Electrical	7	11.86
Tai chi	7	11.86
Prayer	6	10.17
Osteopathic manipulation	5	8.47
Shamanism	5	8.47
Western psychology	4	6.78
Hypnosis	4	6.78
Applied kinesiology	3	5.08
Iridology	2	3.39
Ear candling	2	3.39
Intuitive counseling	2	3.39
Tui na	1	1.69
Aikido	1	1.69
Chakra balancing	1	1.69
Past-life regressions	1	1.69
Tibetan medicine	0	0.00

2. Please rank (with "1" being the most important) the reasons why you chose the modalities at your CAM program:

	Choice 1	Choice 2	Choice 3	Total	Percent
Owner's personal choices	39	5	2	46	79.31
Traditional scientific efficacy	11	9	4	24	41.38
Client/patient safety	2	12	8	22	37.93
Relaxing quality of modality	4	9	6	19	32.76
Self-conducted market research	1	1	5	7	12.07
Income potential of modality	1	0	1	2	3.45
Professional market research	0	1	1	2	3.45

3. What is the most frequent way in which patients/clients are referred to your clinic? (Please select only one)

	Number	Percent
Self-referred, word-of-mouth	49	83.05
Self-referred, advertising	6	10.17
Self-referred, phone book	3	5.08
Doctors	1	1.69
Nurses	0	0.00
Other CAM practitioners	0	0.00
Hospitals	0	0.00

	Number	Percent

4. What criteria do you use to select practitioners for your CAM program? (Please check all that apply)

	Number	Percent
Personal choice of self/other practitioners	32	54.24
Licensing (if required)	30	50.85
Appropriate education	24	40.68
Professional affiliation	15	25.42
Client recommendation	11	18.64
Years in practice	10	16.95
No special criteria	2	3.39

5. What is your organizational structure? (Please check all that apply)

	Number	Percent
For profit	34	57.63
Loosely structured practitioner paying rent	19	32.20
MD- or DO-supervised	10	16.95
Nonprofit	7	11.86
Supervised by other medical personnel	5	8.47
No answer	3	5.08
Subprogram of larger organization	2	3.39
Hospital program	1	1.69

6. How do you ascertain client/patient satisfaction?

	Number	Percent
Verbal feedback	53	89.83
Continued growth of business	34	57.63
Written survey	14	23.73
Outside marketing/clinical study	3	5.08

7. What method(s) do you have of ascertaining the effectiveness of your services?

	Number	Percent
Verbal feedback	51	86.44
Continued growth of business	32	54.24
Outside marketing/clinical study	3	5.08
Written survey	2	3.39

8. How do you follow up with your clients?

	Number	Percent
Appointment(s) scheduled	40	67.80
Phone call	24	40.68

	Number	Percent
No specific method	13	22.03
E-mail	12	20.34
Postal service	4	6.78

9. Do you sell nutritional supplements, herbs, natural foods, or other products?

	Number	Percent
Yes	41	69.49
No	12	20.34
No answer	6	10.17

10. What products do you sell? (Please check all that apply)

	Number	Percent
Vitamins/nutraceuticals	32	54.24
Herbs	28	47.46
Homeopathics	21	35.59
Books	18	30.51
Equipment (i.e., neti pots, yoga mats, etc.)	14	23.73
CDs/tapes	9	15.25
Beauty	9	15.25
Packaged food/drink	5	8.47
Fresh food/drink	2	3.39

One sold products from all categories

11. What percentage of your business is product sales?

Of those answering "yes" to question 9, eight did not report a percentage. Of those reporting a percentage, the average was 21.27 percent. The range was 1 percent to 90 percent. Four people reported that product sales accounted for more than half of their revenue.

12. What product generates the highest revenue?

Overwhelmingly, nutritional supplements, including herbs, accounted for highest product revenue.

13. Please rank the popularity of the modalities from question 1 from most popular (1) to least used or demanded. (Please select a maximum of seven):

	Choice 1	Choice 2	Choice 3	Total	Percent
Massage	11	7	3	21	36.21
Diet/nutrition	2	6	11	19	32.76

	Choice 1	Choice 2	Choice 3	Total	Percent
Chiropractic	14	2	1	17	29.31
Chinese medicine	7	5	3	15	25.86
Homeopathy	2	7	1	10	17.24
Meditation	2	2	4	8	13.79
Reiki	2	6	0	8	13.79
Yoga	1	3	4	8	13.79
Naturopathy	1	3	1	5	8.62
Nutraceutical	1	1	3	5	8.62
Tai chi	1	1	3	5	8.62
Therapeutic touch	0	2	3	5	8.62
Vitamins	3	1	1	5	8.62
Ayurvedic medicine	1	1	1	3	5.17
Chi gung	2	0	1	3	5.17
Art/music therapy	0	0	2	2	3.45
Biofeedback	2	0	0	2	3.45
Herbs	0	2	0	2	3.45
Prayer	1	0	1	2	3.45
Osteopathic manipulation	1	1	0	2	3.45
Reflexology	0	1	0	1	1.72
Shamanism	0	1	0	1	1.72
Tibetan medicine	0	0	0	0	0.00

14. What do you consider to be the biggest impediment to the continued growth of complementary and alternative health practices? (Please choose only one)

	Number	Percent
Lack of insurance coverage	23	38.98
Public confusion over CAM	13	22.03
Medical acceptance of CAM	7	11.86
Public acceptance of CAM	4	6.78
Lack of effectiveness of CAM practices	2	3.39
Competition from medical care	2	3.39
Lack of quality in education/oversight	2	3.39
Lack of licensing for modalities	1	1.69

15. Do you accept insurance?

Yes	35	59.32
No	22	37.29
No answer	2	3.39

	Number	Percent
16. For which modalities do you accept insurance? (Select all that apply)		
Chiropractic	15	25.42
Massage	12	20.34
Chinese medicine	4	6.78
Diet/nutrition	4	6.78
Homeopathy	3	5.08
Biofeedback	2	3.39
Herbs	2	3.39
Therapeutic touch	2	3.39
Osteopathic manipulation	2	3.30
Nutraceutical	1	1.69
Chi gung	1	1.69
Reflexology	1	1.69
Reiki	1	1.69
Tai chi	1	1.69
Art/music therapy	0	0.00
Ayurvedic medicine	0	0.00
Meditation	0	0.00
Naturopathy	0	0.00
Prayer	0	0.00
Shamanism	0	0.00
Tibetan medicine	0	0.00
Vitamins	0	0.00
Yoga	0	0.00

17. On a scale of one to ten, with ten being the most important, how important do you consider the ability to accept health insurance in the ability to offer CAM programs?

The answers covered the gamut of one to ten. Thirty-six people (61 percent) said it was of greater than average (5) importance with an average ascribed importance of 6.49 percent. Fourteen people (24 percent) said it was of greatest importance (10).

Appendix D

Health Assessment Tools

The health assessment tools include forms for health assessment, initial practitioner recommendations, and client/patient health plan.

Health Assessment

The three things to remember when working on health issues:

- We can heal, in body, mind, and spirit, but we do not always heal our bodies fully. Our physical world includes entropy and the breakdown of physical structures . . .
- Professionals can help you heal, but the power to do so comes from within you!
- Healing takes time!

Directions: Please complete this form initially on your own and then in conjunction with your health care practitioner. Take several days to think about answers. If you are uncertain as to how to answer any questions, please contact the health care provider who gave you this form. All your answers are confidential and will not be shared with other parties without your consent.

Today's Date _____ Date of Birth _____ Age _____

Place of Birth _____

Last Name _____ First Name _____ Middle _____

Address _____

Address Line 2 _____

City _____ State _____ Zip _____

Home Phone _____ Cell Phone _____

Work Phone _____

Fax _____ E-mail _____

Name of Employer _____

Address of Employer _____

Highest Level of Education Completed _____

Sex   M   F   Height _____ Weight _____ lbs.

Marital/Partner Status _____ No. years _____

How did you find out about our program (referred by)? _____

Primary Care Physician _____ Date of last exam _____

May we contact your physician? _____

Health Insurance Company _____ I.D. # (S.S.#) _____

Group No. _____ Medicaid # _____

Children?

Name   DOB

_____   _____

_____   _____

_____   _____

_____   _____

_____   _____

(List on reverse if necessary)

1. Is there a prediagnosed condition for which you are seeking complementary care?

   a. If so, what is it? _____
   b. When were you diagnosed with this condition? _____
   c. Name of physician or psychology worker who made this diagnosis:
      _____
   d. What tests were done to confirm this diagnosis? _____
      _____
   e. When were these tests done? _____
   f. What was the date and type of the last treatment you received for this condition?
      Date _____ Treatment _____
      _____

For questions 2, 3 and 4, bring the medications, vitamins, and herbs with you if you are not sure how to accurately and completely fill out this section.

2. List medications

Name	Condition	Dosage	Frequency
E.g.: aspirin	recurrent headaches	two 325 mg tablets	as needed

(List on reverse if necessary)

3. List vitamins/nutraceuticals

Name	Condition	Dosage	Frequency
E.g.: CoQ10	heart	two 30 mg tablets	twice daily

(List on reverse if necessary)

4. List herbal remedies

Name	Condition	Dosage	Frequency
E.g.: Black cohosh	change of life	4 gelcaps	2 × per day

(List additional items below if necessary)

5. What are all the things (food, drink, inhaled) that you have consumed in the last 24 hours? *Include all snacks, alcohol, caffeine drinks, and smoking times.*

Please circle:

Do you   Smoke   Drink Alcohol   Use Illegal Substances

List Foods, Alcohol, Caffeine, Smoking (include food combinations)	Quantity	Freshness/ Nutrient Content	How Prepared or Cooked	Spicing	Circumstance or Attitude While Eating (rushed, relaxed, etc.)
Morning					

Snack					
Noon					
Snack					
Evening					
Snack					

6. If applicable, when did you exercise in the last 24 hours (i.e., 3 hours before, or 1 hour after eating)?

   a. What was your exercise in the last 24 hours?

   <u>Activity</u>   <u>Duration</u>   <u>Time of Day</u>

   b. What exercise/physical activity is your normal routine?

   <u>Activity</u>   <u>Times per week</u>   <u>Time of Day</u>   <u>Duration</u>

7. What concerns you most about your health?

8. This area is to be filled in by your health care practitioner—List the constitutional or mind/body type as per a discipline such as Chinese medicine, Ayurveda, or homeopathy:

9. Why are you seeking help from our clinic?

10. In your own words, describe your health complaints:

Problem	Describe	Location, if applies
E.g.: Leg pain	Grabbing, then burning pain	Left calf
E.g.: Feelings of extreme fear and anxiety.	For no reason, a sudden and overwhelming feeling of fear occurs.	

11. What would you most like to achieve with your health? (State a realistic goal)

12. Please describe your daily activities

Wake time: Bed time:
Work hours and activities:

Home activities and housework (chores, projects):

Family responsibilities (transporting children, ill parents, etc.):

13. On the following chart, please list "C" for a current health problem, "P" for a past health problem, and "S" for those problems you suspect.

Abdominal distention

Abortion

Acidity

Addiction

Anemia

Anger, impatience

Anorexia

Anxiety

Arteriosclerosis

Arthritis

Asthma

Awaken unable to breathe

Black stool

Bleeding

Bloat/gain before men-
struation

Blood

Blood clots in menstrua-
tion

Blood in stool

Blurred vision

Bones

Breathing difficulty

Bronchitis

Burning on urination

Calf cramping during
exercise

Cancer

Cardiovascular/heart

Changes in skin color,
or mole size

Cholesterol

Colic/abdominal pain

Colon

Congenital heart

Constipation

Convulsions

Coughing

Coughing up blood

Diabetes

Diarrhea

Discharge from nipples

Discolored phlegm

Earaches

Ears

Edema

Emotional

Emphysema

Environmental allergy

Epilepsy

Epstein-Barr virus

Excessive yellow stool

Excessive menstruation

Eyes

Fainting

Faintness/lightheaded

Fullness beneath breast

Female reproductive

Fever

Fingers and toes bluish

Fingers/toes cold and
numb

Food allergies

Frequent burping

Frequent colds

Frequent crying

Frequent urination

Gallbladder

Gastrointestinal

Get up to urinate

Goiter

Gout

Hay fever

Head

Headaches/migraines

Heart attack

Heartburn

Heavy menstrual flow

Hemorrhoids

Hepatitis

Hernia

High blood pressure

HIV/AIDS

Hot flashes

Hyperthyroid

Hypothyroid

Immune system

Indigestion

Irregular menstruation

Irregular or rapid heart-
beat

Jaundice

Joint pain

Kidney

Lethargy

Leukemia

Liver

Urinate while cough-
ing/sneezing

Low blood pressure

Lower back pain

Lumps in breast

Lumps in testicles

Male reproductive

Memory trouble

Menopause

Menstruation before 10

Menstruation after 15

Mental health

Menstrual trouble

Metabolic/endocrine

Migraine

Miscarriage

Mouth

Muscles

Nasal stuffiness

Nausea (frequent)

Nervous breakdown

Nervous system

Night sweats

Nose

Other congenital illness

Overweight

Pain in chest

Pain in legs or feet

Pain, where:

Parasites

Pass a lot of gas

PMS

Poor appetite

Poor night vision

Post nasal drainage

Prostate

Rectum

Respiratory

Rheumatic heart

Rheumatism

Ringing in ears

Sinus	Trouble hearing	Used birth control, type:
Sinus Infection	Trouble speaking/getting	Vomit blood
Skin disorder	words out	Vomiting
Small intestine	Trouble swallowing	Wheezing
Sore or bleeding gums	Tuberculosis	Worry, fear, nervous
Sore throat	Tumors	
Stomach	Ulcers	
Stroke	Unhealed wounds,	
Suicide thoughts	where:	
Swollen feet or ankles	Upper-back pain	
Throat	Urine	
Tightness in chest	Urine leaking	

14. List Allergies/Sensitivities

    Medication:

    Food:

    Inhalant: (e.g., molds, pets, pollen)

    Skin: (e.g., wool, latex)

    My sinus/allergies are:
    1. worse indoors in the winter; 2. worse outdoors in spring and summer; or 3. always bad.

15. Family History:

Name	Age	Health	Age at Death	Cause of Death
Mother				
Father				
Brothers/Sisters (indicate which) 1.				
2.				
3.				
4.				
5.				
Spouse/Partner				

Sons/Daughters (indicate which) 1.				
2.				
3.				
4.				
5.				
Maternal Grandmother				
Maternal Grandfather				
Paternal Grandmother				
Paternal Grandfather				

16. Have you or any family members ever had any addictions (i.e., drugs, alcohol, other)? If so, what, and who?

17. Have you ever been physically or emotionally abused (as a child, from family members, at work, at school)?

18. Describe areas of psychological stress in your life:

19. Was there a traumatic event in your life one or two years ago (e.g., loss of loved one, job, violence)?

20. What events are coming up in your life that might cause apprehension?

21. Please answer the following questions by circling always, usually, sometimes, rarely, or never:

Emotional life:

a. I feel good about myself.

Always   Usually   Sometimes   Rarely   Never

b. I can release negative emotions.

Always   Usually   Sometimes   Rarely   Never

c. I am able to give love.

Always   Usually   Sometimes   Rarely   Never

d. I am able to receive love.

Always   Usually   Sometimes   Rarely   Never

e. My sleep is restful.

Always   Usually   Sometimes   Rarely   Never

f. I accept my sexual desires.

Always   Usually   Sometimes   Rarely   Never

g. I accept it if I get angry, fearful, or depressed.

Always   Usually   Sometimes   Rarely   Never

h. I embrace life.

Always   Usually   Sometimes   Rarely   Never

i. I can share my feelings with friends or family.

Always   Usually   Sometimes   Rarely   Never

j. I accept constructive criticism.

Always   Usually   Sometimes   Rarely   Never

k. I can say "no" to demands that overextend me.

Always   Usually   Sometimes   Rarely   Never

l. I can spend happy time alone.

Always   Usually   Sometimes   Rarely   Never

m. I can talk about death.

Always   Usually   Sometimes   Rarely   Never

n. I am happy with my family.

Always   Usually   Sometimes   Rarely   Never

o. I am happy with my friends.

    Always   Usually   Sometimes   Rarely   Never

p. I am happy with my spouse.

    Always   Usually   Sometimes   Rarely   Never

q. I love my family and friends.

    Always   Usually   Sometimes   Rarely   Never

Work:

r. I love my job.

    Always   Usually   Sometimes   Rarely   Never

s. My job equals my well-being.

    Always   Usually   Sometimes   Rarely   Never

t. I have low stress in my work.

    Always   Usually   Sometimes   Rarely   Never

u. I have authority to do my job.

    Always   Usually   Sometimes   Rarely   Never

v. I get along with my boss.

    Always   Usually   Sometimes   Rarely   Never

w. I get along with my co-workers.

    Always   Usually   Sometimes   Rarely   Never

x. I am good at my job.

    Always   Usually   Sometimes   Rarely   Never

22. Please circle the answer that best describes you for each row of three across:

Atheistic	Spiritual	Agnostic
Punishment	Forgiveness	Justice
Lack enthusiasm	Enthusiastic	Excitable
Lack creativity	Creative	Overfantasize
Low energy	Energetic	Nervous/jittery
Hate details	Concise	Fastidious
Poor communicator	Good communicator	Overly talkative

Don't understand religion	Spiritual ideals are logical	I am angry with God
Prevention doesn't work	Prevention can work	Revenge first
Disinterested	Curious	Nosy
Often confused	Clear headed	Critical
Trouble thinking	Concentrate well	Have headaches
Fearsome	Courageous	Foolhardy
Accepting of all	Stand up for rights	Prove my point
Good and evil are the same	Loving	Sentimental
Apathetic	Love despite faults	Love begets forgiveness
Impatient	Patient	Passive
Discontent	Content	Lethargic
Get sick often	Strong immunity	Never know when I'm ill
Tired	Good endurance	Don't feel pain

23. Please answer the following questions about your spiritual/religious pursuits

   a. Do you belong to a group, synagogue, church, mosque, etc., that shares spiritual explorations?
   If so, which religion/organization? _____

   b. Do you have similar or conflicting views on spirituality and/or religious pursuits as your family and friends? _____

   c. Would you say your place of worship was more political or spiritual? _____

   d. True or False: Spirituality flows from an external "God" force.

   e. True or False: Spirituality comes from within.

   f. True or False: It is easy for me to forgive and let go of things.

   g. Rank these statements from most (1) to least (3) in how they apply to you:
   _____ Learn from the past
   _____ Live for today
   _____ Plan for the future

   h. True or False: I am more important than the people and things around me.

   i. In your own words, describe how you are connected to the sun:
   _____
   _____
   _____

Initial Practitioner Recommendations

Date: _____ Client Name: _____

Diet:

Environment:

Exercise/Activities:

Hygiene:

Herbs/Nutraceuticals:

Affirmations (NLP):

Referrals (Physicians, tests, other practitioners):

A second set of recommendations from a team of health care providers will be made by: _____ (date)

These suggestions are for the improvement of health and do not diagnose, treat, or attempt to cure any disease.

Client/Patient Health Plan

Client Name and Identifying No. _____

Date of clinic team meeting: _____ Practitioners: _____

_____

Buddy: _____

Risk Factors and Plan

Causes

Internal

    Physiological

    Plan to reduce:

    Psychological

    Plan to reduce:

External

    Physiological

    Plan to reduce:

    Psychosocial

    Plan to reduce:

Client/Patient Health Plan
Page 2

Risk Factors and Plan

Triggers (Primary Prevention Issues)

Internal

    Physiological

    Plan to reduce:

    Psychospiritual

    Plan to reduce:

External

    Physiological

    Plan to reduce:

    Psychological

    Plan to reduce:

I understand this plan, and understand that it is shared with practitioners, and my buddy/mentor. I will work to achieve these goals over the next year:

_____   _____

Client/Patient   Date

Bibliography

Agnihotri, S. and Vaidya, A.D. (1996). A novel approach to study antibacterial properties of volatile components of selected Indian medicinal herbs. *Indian Journal of Experimental Biology*, 34 (7), 712-715.

Alam, M., Susan, T., Joy, S. and Kundu, A.B. (1992). Antiinflammatory and antipyretic activity of vicolides of *Vicoa indica* DC. *Indian Journal of Experimental Biology*, 30 (1), 38-41.

Almond, B.J. (1997). Magnet therapy reduces pain in post-polio patients. *Texas Medical Center News*, 19 (23).

An alternative medicine treatment for Parkinson's disease: Results of a multicenter clinical trial (1995). *Journal of Alternative and Complementary Medicine*, 1 (3), 249-255.

Arjungi, K.N. (1976). Areca nut: A review. *Arzneimittelforschung*, 26 (5), 951-956.

Astin, J.A., Ariane, M., Pelletier, K.R., Hansen, E. and Haskell, W.L. (1998). A review of the incorporation of complementary and alternative medicine by mainstream physicians. *JAMA*, 158 (21), 2303-2310.

Astin, J.A., Harkness, E. and Ernst, E. (2000). The efficacy of "distant healing": A systematic review of randomized trials. *Annals of Internal Medicine*, 6 (132), 903-910.

Atal, C.K., Zutshi, U. and Rao, P.G. (1981). Scientific evidence on the role of Ayurvedic herbals on bioavailability of drugs. *Journal of Ethnopharmacology*, 4 (2), 229-232.

Baerheim, A., Algroy, R., Skogedal, K.R., Stephansen, R. and Sandvik, H. (1998). Feet—a diagnostic tool? *Tidsskr Nor Laegeforen*, 118 (5), 753-755.

Bajaj, S. and Vohora, S.B. (1998). Analgesic activity of gold preparations used in Ayurveda and Unani-Tibb. *Indian Journal of Medical Research*, (108), 104-111.

Bapat, R.D., Acharya, B.S., Juvekar, S. and Dahanukar, S.A. (1998). Leech therapy for complicated varicose veins. *Indian Journal of Medical Research*, (107), 281-284.

Bhattacharya, A., Ramanathan, M., Ghosal, S. and Bhattacharya, S.K. (2000). Effect of withania somnifera glycowithanolides on iron-induced hepatotoxicity in rats. *Phytotherapy Research*, 14 (7), 568-570.

Bhattacharya, S.K., Bhattacharya, A. and Chakrabarti, A. (2000). Adaptogenic activity of Siotone, a polyherbal formulation of Ayurvedic rasayanas. *Indian Journal of Experimental Biology*, 38 (2), 119-128.

Bhattacharya, S.K., Bhattacharya, A., Sairam, K. and Ghosal, S. (2000). Anxioly-tic-antidepressant activity of withania somnifera glycowithanolides: An experi-mental study. *Phytomedicine*, 7 (6), 463-469.

Bhattacharya, S.K. and Kumar, A. (1997). Effect of trasina, an Ayurvedic herbal formulation, on experimental models of Alzheimer's disease and central choli-nergic markers in rats. *Journal of Alternative and Complementary Medicine*, 3 (4), 327-336.

Bhide, S.V. and Lubri, A. (1997). Effect of turmeric oil and turmeric oleoresin on cytogenetic damage in patients suffering from oral submucous fibrosis. *Cancer Lett*, 116 (2), 265-269.

Buchbauer, G., Jirovetz, L., Jager, W., Dietrich, H. and Plank, C. (1991). Aroma-therapy: Evidence for sedative effects of the essential oil of lavender after inhala-tion. *Zeitschrift für Naturforschung*, 46 (1112), 1067-1072.

Buchbauer, G., Jirovetz, L., Jager, W., Plank, C. and Dietrich, H. (1993). Fragrance compounds and essential oils with sedative effects upon inhalation. *Journal of Pharmacological Science*, 82 (6), 660-664.

Buckle, J. (1993). Aromatherapy. *Nursing Times*, 89 (20), 32-35.

Burkhart, C.G., Weintraub, M.I., Blechman, A.M. and Jonas, S. (2000). Letters to the editor section: Use of magnets. *JAMA*. 284 (5), (Online). Available: <http://jama.ama-assn.org/issues/v284n5/ffull/jlt0802-4.html>.

Burkhart, M.A. (2000). Healing relationships with nature. *Complementary Therapy in Nursing and Midwifery*, 6 (1), 35-40.

Cannard, G. (1996). The effect of aromatherapy in promoting relaxation and stress reduction in a general hospital. *Complementary Therapy and Nursing Mid-wifery*, 2 (2), 38-40.

Cassileth, B.R. (1998). *The Alternative Medicine Handbook: The Complete Refer-ence Guide to Alternative and Complementary Therapies*. New York: W. W. Norton and Company.

Cawthorn, A. (1995). A review of the literature surrounding the research into aro-matherapy. *Complementary Therapy and Nursing Midwifery*, 1 (4), 118-120.

Ching, M. (1999). Contemporary therapy: Aromatherapy in the management of acute pain? *Contemporary Nursing*, 8 (4), 146-151.

Chopra, D. (1991). *Unconditional Life*. New York: HarperCollins Publishers.

Chopra, D. (1993). *Ageless Body, Timeless Mind*. New York: Harmony Books.

Clendenin, M. (2000). Intergrative medicine: Open to a wider world. *Jefferson Medical College Alumni Bulletin*, 49 (2), 5.

Collacott, E.A., Zimmerman, J.T., White, D.W., Rindone, J.P. and Pharm, D. (2000). Bipolar permanent magnets for the treatment of chronic low back pain. *JAMA*, 283 (10), 1322-1325.

Cooke, B. and Ernst, E. (2000). Aromatherapy: A systematic review. *British Jour-nal of General Practice*, 50 (455), 493-496.

Council for Scientific Affairs (2001). *Alternative Medicine Report* 12. Chicago: American Medical Association.

Cox, C.L. and Hayes, J.A. (1997). Reducing anxiety: The employment of therapeutic touch as a nursing intervention. *Complementary Therapy and Nursing Midwifery,* 3 (6), 163-167.

Cox, C. and Hayes, J. (1999). Physiologic and psychodynamic responses to the administration of therapeutic touch in critical care. *Complementary Therapy and Nursing Midwifery,* 5 (3), 87-92.

Crane, B. (1998). *Reflexology.* New York: Barnes & Noble Books.

Dale, A. and Cornwell, S. (1994). The role of lavender oil in relieving perineal discomfort following childbirth: A blind randomized clinical trial. *Journal of Advanced Nursing,* 19 (1), 89-96.

Daley, B. (1998). Therapeutic touch, nursing practice and contemporary cutaneous wound healing research. *Journal of Advanced Nursing,* 25 (6), 1123-1132.

Dalvi, S.S., Nadkarni, P.M. and Gupta, K.C. (1990). Effect of *Asparagus racemosus* (Shatavari) on gastric emptying time in normal healthy volunteers. *Journal of Postgraduate Medicine,* 36 (2), 91-94.

Degan, M., Fabris, F., Vanin, F., Bevilacqua, M. and Genova, V. (2000). The effectiveness of foot reflexotherapy on chronic pain associated with a herniated disk. *Professioni Infermieristiche,* 53 (2), 80-87.

Dev, S. (1999). Ancient-modern concordance in Ayurvedic plants: Some examples. *Environmental Health Perspective,* 107 (10), 783-789.

Diego, M.A., Jones, N.A., Field, T., Hernandez-Reif, M., Schanberg, S., Kuhn, C., McAdam, V., Galamaga, R. and Galamaga, M. (1998). Aromatherapy positively affects mood, EEG patterns of alertness and math computations. *International Journal of Neuroscience,* 96 (34), 217-224.

Dossey, L. (1999). *Reinventing Medicine.* New York: HarperCollins Publishers.

Drug company expected to pay $840 million fine. (2001). *Morning Call,* May 29, p. A5.

Dunn, C., Sleep, J. and Collett, D. (1995). Sensing an improvement: An experimental study to evaluate the use of aromatherapy, massage and periods of rest in an intensive care unit. *Journal of Advanced Nursing,* 21 (2), 34-40.

Dyer, W. W. (1995). *Your Sacred Self.* New York: HarperCollins Publishers.

Easter, A. (1997). The state of research on the effects of therapeutic touch. *Journal of Holistic Nursing,* 15 (2), 158-175.

Eckes Peck, S.D. (1997). The effectiveness of therapeutic touch for decreasing pain in elders with degenerative arthritis. *Journal of Holistic Nursing,* 15 (2), 176-198.

Ernst, E. and White, A.R. (1998). Acupuncture for back pain: A meta-analysis of randomized controlled trials. *Archives of Internal Medicine,* 158 (20), 2235-2241.

Frawley, D. (1988). *The Yoga of Herbs.* Twin Lakes, WI: Lotus Press.

Frawley, D. (1989). *Ayurvedic Healing.* Salt Lake City, UT: Morton Publishing.

Frawley, D. (1994). *Tantric Yoga and the Wisdom Goddesses.* Salt Lake City, UT: Morton Publishing.

Frawley, D. (1996). *Ayurveda and the Mind.* Twin Lakes, WI: Lotus Press.

Fujiwara, R., Komori, T., Noda, Y., Kuraoka, T. and Shibata, H. (1998). Effects of a long-term inhalation of fragrances on the stress-induced immunosuppression in mice. *Neuroimmunomodulation*, 5 (6), 318-322.

Garfinkle, M., Singhal, A., Katz, W. and Allan, D. (1998). Yoga-based intervention for carpal tunnel syndrome: A randomized trial. *JAMA* (280), 1601-1603.

General Accounting Office (U.S.) (2000). Adverse drug events (Online). Available: <http://www.gao.gov> (search by GAO/HEHS-00-21).

Giasson, M. and Bouchard, L. (1998). Effect of therapeutic touch on the well-being of persons with terminal cancer. *Journal of Holistic Nursing*, 16 (3), 383-398.

Giasson, M., Leroux, G., Tardif, H. and Bouchard, L. (1999). Therapeutic touch (French). *L'Infirmière du Québec*, 6 (6), 38-47.

Goldberg, S. (1999). *Clinical Biochemistry Made Ridiculously Simple*. Miami, FL: MedMaster, Inc.

Gordon, A., Merenstein, J.H., D'Amico, F. and Hudgens, D. (1998). The effects of therapeutic touch on patients with osteoarthritis of the knee. *Journal of Family Practice*, 47 (4), 271-277.

Hay, I.C., Jamieson, M. and Oremerod, A.D. (1999). Randomized trial of aromatherapy: Successful treatment for alopecia areata. *Archives of Dermatology*, November (134), 11.

Hay, L.L. (1987). *You Can Heal Your Life*. Carlsbad, CA: Hay House, Inc.

Heidt, P. (1981). Effect of therapeutic touch on anxiety level of hospitalized patients. *Nursing Research*, 30 (1), 32-37.

Hinman, A. and Richards, A. (1998). Fourth-grade science project casts doubt on "therapeutic touch" (Online). Available: <http://www.cnn.com/HEALTH/9804/01/therapeutic.touch/>.

Hoffmann, D. (1992). *The New Holistic Herbal*. Rockport, MA: Element Books Limited.

Hrobjartsson, A. and Gotzsche, C. (2001). Is the placebo powerless?—An analysis of clinical trials comparing placebo with no treatment. *New England Journal of Medicine*, 344 (21), 1594-1602.

Ilmberger, J., Heuberger, E., Mahrhofer, C., Dessovic, H. and Kowarik, D. (2001). The influence of essential oils on human attention. I: Alertness. *Chemistry of Senses*, 26 (2), 239-245.

Ireland, M. (1998). Therapeutic touch with HIV-infected children: A pilot study. *Journal of the Association of Nurses in AIDS Care*, 9 (4), 68-77.

Ireland, M. and Olson, M. (2000). Massage therapy and therapeutic touch in children: State of the science. *Alternative Therapy Health and Medicine*, 6 (5), 54-63.

Itai, T., Amayasu, H., Kuribayashi, M., Kawamura, N. and Okada, M. (2000). Psychological effects of aromatherapy on chronic hemodialysis patients. *Psychiatry and Clinical Neuroscience*, 54 (4), 393-397.

Johnson, L.A. (2001). Study scoffs at placebo effect. *The Morning Call*, May 24, p. A9.

Jones, S.S. (1992). *Choose to Live Peacefully.* Berkeley, CA: Celestial Arts Publishing.

Journal of the American Medical Association (JAMA) (2001). Acupuncture search. *JAMA.* Database search, Chicago (Online). Available: <http://www.ama-assn. org/cgi-bin/search?T=results.hts&C=25&S=1&QueryText=acupuncture& M=I &collection=public&collection=members&collection=publishing&collection =&x =41&y=27>.

Keegan, L. (2001). *Healing with Complementary and Alternative Therapies.* Albany, NY: Delmar.

Keller, E. and Bzdek, V.M. (1986). Effects of therapeutic touch on tension headache pain. *Nursing Research,* 35 (2), 101-106.

Kesselring, A. (1994). Foot reflex zone massage. *Schweizeriche Medizinische Wochenschrift Supplementum,* (62), 88-93.

Kesselring, A. (1999). Foot reflexology massage: A clinical study. *Forsch Komplementarmed,* 6 (1), 38-40.

Kesselring, A., Spichiger, E. and Muller, M. (1998). Foot reflexology: An intervention study. *Pflegeforschung,* 11 (4), 213-218.

Kilstoff, K. and Chenoweth, L. (1998). New approaches to health and well-being for dementia day-care clients, family carers and day-care staff. *International Journal of Nursing Practice,* 4 (2), 70-83.

Kirschmann, G. and Kirschmann, J. (1996). *Nutrition Almanac.* New York: McGraw-Hill.

Kite, S.M., Maher, E.J., Anderson, K., Young, T. and Young, J. (1998). Development of an aromatherapy service at a cancer centre. *Palliative Medicine,* 12 (3), 171-180.

Kramer, N.A. (1990). Comparison of therapeutic touch and casual touch in stress reduction of hospitalized children. *Pediatric Nursing,* 16 (5), 483-485.

La Torre, D. (2001). Insurance bitter pill for doctors to swallow. *Morning Call,* May 29, pp. A1, A5.

Labadie, R.P. and Woerdenbag, A. (1995). Ayurvedic herbal drugs with possible cytostatic activity. *Journal of Ethnopharmacology,* 47 (2), 75-84.

Lafreniere, K.D., Mutus, B., Cameron, S., Tannous, M. and Giannotti, M. (1999). Effects of therapeutic touch on biochemical and mood indicators in women. *Journal of Alternative and Complementary Medicine,* 5 (4), 367-370.

Lazarou, J., Pomeranz, B.H. and Corey, P.N. (1998). Incidence of adverse drug reactions in hospitalized patients: A meta-analysis of prospective studies. *Journal of the American Medical Association,* 279, 1200-1205.

Lee, K.G., Mitchell, A. and Shibamoto, T. (2000). Antioxidative activities of aroma extracts isolated from natural plants. *Biofactors,* 13 (14), 173-178.

Lis-Balchin, M., Deans, S. and Hart, S. (1997). A study of the changes in the bioactivity of essential oils used singly and as mixtures in aromatherapy. *Journal of Alternative and Complementary Medicine,* 3 (3), 249-256.

Lis-Balchin, M. and Hart, S. (1999). Studies on the mode of action of the essential oil of lavender (*Lavandula angustifolia* P. Miller). *Phytotherapy Research*, 13 (6), 540-542.

Lis-Balchin, M., Hart S.L. and Deans, S.G. (2000). Pharmacological and antimicrobial studies on different tea-tree oils (*Melaleuca alternifolia, Leptospermum scoparium* or Manuka and *Kunzea ericoides* or Kanuka), originating in Australia and New Zealand. *Phytotherapy Research*, 14 (8), 623-629.

Lohda, R. and Bagga, A. (2000). Traditional Indian systems of medicine. *Annals of Academic Medicine Singapore*, 29 (1), 37-41.

Meehan, T.C. (1993). Therapeutic touch and postoperative pain: A Rogerian research study. *Nursing Science Quarterly*, 6 (2), 69-78.

Melchart, D., Linde, K., Fischer, P., White, A., Allais, G., Vickers, A. and Berman, B. (1999). Acupuncture for recurrent headaches: A systematic review of randomized controlled trials. *Cephalalgia*, 19 (9), 779-786.

Misra, R. (1998). Modern drug development from traditional medicinal plants using radioligand receptor-binding assays. *Medicine Research Review*, 18 (5), 383-402.

Nagashayana, N., Sankarankutty, P., Nampoothiri, M.R., Mohan, P.K. and Mohanakumar, K.P. (2000). Association of L-DOPA with recovery following Ayurveda medication in Parkinson's disease. *Journal of Neurological Science*, (176), 124-127.

National Institute of Health (1997). NIH Panel Issues Consensus Statement on Acupuncture. NIH News Release. (Online). Available: <http://www.nih.gov/news/pr/nov97/od-05.htm>.

Oleson, T. and Flocco, W. (1993). Randomized controlled study of premenstrual symptoms treated with ear, hand, and foot reflexology. *Obstetrics and Gynecology*, 82 (6), 906-911.

Olson, K. and Hanson, J. (1997). Using Reiki to manage pain: A preliminary report. *Cancer Prevention Control*, 1 (2), 108-113.

Olson, M., Sneed, N., Bonadonna, R., Ratliff, J. and Dias, J. (1992). Therapeutic touch and post-Hurricane Hugo stress. *Journal of Holistic Nursing*, 10 (2), 120-136.

Olson, M., Sneed, N., LaVia, M., Virella, G. and Bonadonna, R. (1997). Stress-induced immunosuppression and therapeutic touch. *Alternative Therapies in Health and Medicine*, 3 (2), 68-74.

Ornish, D., Shwerwitz, L.W., Billings, J.H., Brown, S.E., Gould, K.L., Merritt, T.A., Sparler, S., Armstrong, W.T., Ports, T.A., Kirkeeide, R.I., Hogeboom, C. and Brand, R.J. (1998). Intensive lifestyle changes for reversal of coronary artery disease. *Journal of the American Medical Association*, 280, 2001-2007.

Papadopoulos, A., Wright, S. and Ensor, J. (1999). Evaluation and attributional analysis of an aromatherapy service for older adults with physical health problems and carers using the service. *Complementary Therapy Medicine*, 7 (4), 239-244.

Patel, M., Gutzwiller, F., Paccaud, F. and Marazzi, A. (1989). A meta-analysis of acupuncture for chronic pain. *International Journal of Epidemiology,* 18 (4), 900-906.

Patil, S., Kanase, A. and Kulkarni, P.H. (2000). Antianaemic properties of ayurvedic drugs, raktavardhak, punarnavasav and navayas louh in albino rats during phenylhydrazine induced haemolytic anaemia. *Indian Journal of Experimental Biology,* 38 (3), 253-257.

Peck, S.D. (1998). The efficacy of therapeutic touch for improving functional ability in elders with degenerative arthritis. *Nursing Science Quarterly,* 11 (3), 123-132.

Pohocha, N. and Grampurohit, N. (2001). Antispasmodic activity of the fruits of *Helicteres isora* Linn. *Phytotherapy Research,* 15 (1), 49-52.

Ramanoelina, A.R., Terrom, G.P., Bianchini, J.P. and Coulanges, P. (1987). Antibacterial action of essential oils extracted from Madagascar plants. *Archives de l'Institut Pasteur de Madagascar,* 53 (1), 217-226.

Ramanujam, S., Shanmugasundaram, K.R. and Shanmugasundaram, E.R. (1994). Amrita Bindu—a salt-spice-herbal health food supplement for the prevention of nitrosamine induced depletion of antioxidants. *Journal of Ethnopharmacology,* 42 (2), 83-93.

Rauch, E. (1993). *Diagnostics According to F. X. Mayr.* Brussels, Belgium: Haug International.

Riet, G., Kleijnen, J. and Knipschild, P. (1990). Acupuncture and chronic pain: A criteria-based meta-analysis. *Journal of Clinical Epidemiology,* 43 (11), 1191-1199.

Romine, I.J., Bush, A.M. and Gesit, C.R. (1999). Lavender aromatherapy in recovery from exercise. *Perceptual and Motor Skills,* 88 (31), 756-758.

Rosa, L., Rosa, E., Sarner, L. and Barrett, S. (1998). A close look at therapeutic touch. *Journal of the American Medical Association,* 279, 1005-1010.

Rowser, K. (1999). *Changing the Past.* Lexington Cottage, England: Cathee Courter and Kieran Rowser.

Saeki, Y. (2000). The effect of foot-bath with or without the essential oil of lavender on the autonomic nervous system: A randomized trial. *Complementary Therapy Medicine,* 8 (1), 2-7.

Samarel, N., Fawcett, J., Davis, M.M. and Ryan, F.M. (1998). Effects of dialogue and therapeutic touch on preoperative and postoperative experiences of breast cancer surgery: An exploratory study. *Oncology Nursing Forum,* 25 (8), 1369-1376.

Saraf, M.N., Ghooi, R.B. and Patwardhan, B.K. (1989). Studies on the mechanism of action of *Semecarpus anacardium* in rheumatoid arthritis. *Journal of Ethnopharmacology,* 25 (2), 159-164.

Sayette, M.A. and Parrott, D.J. (1999). Effects of olfactory stimuli on urge reduction in smokers. *Experimental Clinical Psychopharmacology,* 7 (2), 151-159.

Shevrygin, B.V., Fedorova, T.V. and Pekli, F.F. (1999). Natural ether oils in the treatment of chronic pharyngitis in children in pediatric practice. *Vestnik Otorinolaringologii*, (2), 52-53.

Siegel, B. S. (1998). *Peace, Love and Healing*. New York: Harper Perennial.

Singh, R.K., Acharya, S.B. and Bhattacharya, S.K. (2000). Pharmacological activity of *Elaeocarpus sphaericus*. *Phytotherapy Research*, 14 (1), 36-39.

Singh, R.K., Nath, G., Acharya, S.B. and Goel, R.K. (1997). Pharmacological actions of *Pongamia pinnata* roots in albino rats. *Indian Journal of Experimental Biology*, 35 (8), 831-836.

Singh, R.K., Nath, G., Goel, R.K. and Bhattacharya, S.K. (1998). Pharmacological actions of *Abies pindrow* Royle leaf. *Indian Journal of Experimental Biology*, 36 (2), 187-191.

Siurin, S.A. (1997). Effects of essential oil on lipid peroxidation and lipid metabolism in patients with chronic bronchitis. *Klinicheskaia Meditsina*, 75 (10), 43-45.

Smith, D.E. and Salerno, J.W. (1992). Selective growth inhibition of a human malignant melanoma cell line by sesame oil in vitro. *Prostaglandins Leukot Essential Fatty Acids*, 46 (2), 145-150.

Sneed, N.V., Olson, M., Bubolz, B. and Finch, N. (2001). Influences of a relaxation intervention on perceived stress and power spectral analysis of heart rate variability. *Progressive Cardiovascular Nursing*, 16 (2), 57-64, 79.

Spence, J.E. and Olson, M.A. (1997). Quantitative research on therapeutic touch. An integrative review of the literature 1985-1995. *Scandanavian Journal of Caring Science*, 11 (3), 183-190.

Srivastava, K.C. (1989). Extracts from two frequently consumed spices—cumin *(Cuminum cyminum)* and turmeric *(Curcuma longa)*—inhibit platelet aggregation and alter eicosanoid biosynthesis in human blood platelets. *Prostaglandins Leukot Essential Fatty Acids*, 37 (1), 57-64.

Srivastava, K.C., Bordia, A. and Verma, S.K. (1995). Curcumin, a major component of food spice turmeric *(Curcuma longa)* inhibits aggregation and alters eicosanoid metabolism in human blood platelets. *Prostaglandins Leukot Essential Fatty Acids*, 52 (4), 223-227.

Stephenson, N.L., Weinrich, S.P. and Tavakoli, A.S. (2000). The effects of foot reflexology on anxiety and pain in patients with breast and lung cancer. *Oncology Nursing Forum*, 27 (1), 67-72.

Sudmeier, I., Bodner, G., Egger, I., Mur, E. and Ulmer, M. (1999). Changes of renal blood flow during organ-associated foot reflexology measured by color Doppler sonography. *Forsch Komplementarmed*, 6 (3), 129-134.

Sugiura, M., Hayakawa, R., Kato, Y., Sugiura, K. and Hashimoto, R. (2000). Results of patch testing with lavender oil in Japan. *Contact Dermatitis*, 43 (3), 157-160.

Tamhane, M.D., Thorat, S.P., Rege, N.N. and Dahanukar, S.A. (1997). Effect of oral administration of *Terminalia chebula* on gastric emptying: An experimental study. *Journal of Postgraduate Medicine*, 43 (1), 12-13.

Thorat, S.P., Rege, N.N., Naik, A.S., Thatte, U.M. and Joshi, A. (1995). *Emblica officinalis:* A novel therapy for acute pancreatitis—an experimental study. *HPB Surgery,* 9 (1), 25-30.

Tirtha, S.S. (1998). *The Ayurveda Encyclopedia.* Bayville, NY: Ayurveda Holistic Center Press.

Tokar, E. (1998). Tibetan Medicine History. Innovision Communications. (Online). Available: <http://www.tibetanmedicine.com>.

Turner, J.G., Clark A.J., Gauthier, D.K. and Williams, M. (1998). The effect of therapeutic touch on pain and anxiety in burn patients. *Journal of Advanced Nursing,* 28 (1), 10-20.

Ullman, D. (1991). *Discovering Homeopathy.* Berkeley California: North Atlantic Books.

Ullman, D. (1995). *Consumer's Guide to Homeopathy.* (Online). Available: <http://www.homeopathic.com/procare/>.

Ulrich, S. (1998). Fact Sheet for PINPOINT Electronic Drug Profile. Portland, OR Provider Advantage (Online). Available: <http://www.provider-advantage.com/news.html>. Accessed December 2000.

United States Food and Drug Administration (1999). Milestones in U.S. Food and Drug Law History. FDA. Washington, DC (Online). Available: <http://vm.cfsan.fda.gov/mileston.html>.

Verma, V. (1995). *Ayurveda: A Way of Life.* York Beach, ME: Samuel Weiser, Inc.

Vickers, A.J. and Smith, C. (2001). Homeopathic Oscillococcinum for preventing and treating influenza and influenza-like syndromes. *The Cochrane Library.* Oxford, England (Online). Available: <http://www.update-software.com/abstracts/ab001957.htm>.

Walter, G. and Rey, J.M. (1999). The relevance of herbal treatments for psychiatric practice. *Australian New Zealand Journal of Psychiatry,* 33 (4), 482-489.

Wardell, D.W. and Engebretson, J. (2001). Biological correlates of Reiki touch (sm) healing. *Journal of Advanced Nursing,* 33 (4), 439-445.

Weil, A. (1980). *The Marriage of the Sun and the Moon.* Boston: Houghton Mifflin.

Weil, A. (1995). *Health and Healing.* New York: Houghton Mifflin.

Weil, A. (1996). Vitamin C: Aids recovery from surgery? Ask Dr. Weil (Online). Available: <http://www.drweil.com/app/cda/drw_cda.html?command=TodayQA&pt=Question&questionId=4085>.

Weil, A. (1997a). Acceptance of acupuncture? Ask Dr. Weil (Online). Available: <http://www.drweil.com/app/cda/drw_cda.html?command=TodayQA&pt=Question& questionId=3131>.

Weil, A. (1997b). Too many vitamins? Ask Dr. Weil (Online). Available: <http://www.drweil.com/app/cda/drw_cda.html?command=TodayQA&pt=Question& questionId=3113>.

Weil, A. (1999). Electric therapy for lower back pain? Ask Dr. Weil (Online). Available: <http://www.drweil.com/app/cda/drw_cda.html?command=TodayQA&pt =Question&questionId=3577>.

Weil, A. (2001). Vitamin C: Hard on your heart? Ask Dr. Weil (Online). Available: <http://www.drweil.com/app/cda/drw_cda.html?command=TodayQA&pt=Question &questionId=3845>.

Weiss, D.R., Sharma, S.D., Gaur, R.K., Sharma, J.S. and Desai, A. (1986). Traditional concepts of mental disorder among Indian psychiatric patients: Preliminary report of work in progress. *Social Science & Medicine,* 23 (4), 379-386.

Wiebe, E. (2000). A randomized trial of aromatherapy to reduce anxiety before abortion. *Effective Clinical Practice,* 3 (4), 166-169.

Wilkinson, S., Aldridge, J., Salmon, I., Cain, E. and Wilson, B. (1999). An evaluation of aromatherapy massage in palliative care. *Palliative Medicine,* 13 (5), 409-417.

Wilson, L. (1998). *Legal Guidelines for Unlicensed Practitioners.* Prescott, AZ: L. D. Wilson Consultants, Inc.

Winstead-Fry, P. and Kijek, J. (1999). An integrative review and meta-analysis of therapeutic touch research. *Alternative Therapies in Health and Medicine,* 5 (6), 58-67.

Wirth, D.P. (1995). Complementary healing intervention and dermal wound reepithelialization: An overview. *International Journal of Psychosomatics,* 42 (14), 48-53.

Wirth, D.P. and Barrett, M.J. (1994). Complementary healing therapies. *International Journal of Psychosomatic Medicine,* 41 (14), 61-67.

Wirth, D.P. and Cram, J.R. (1993). Multi-site electromyographic analysis of non-contact therapeutic touch. *International Journal of Psychosomatics,* 40 (14), 47-55.

Wirth, D.P. and Cram, J.R. (1994). The psychophysiology of nontraditional prayer. *International Journal of Psychosomatics,* 41 (14), 68-75.

Wirth, D.P., Cram, J.R. and Chang, R.J. (1997). Multisite electromyographic analysis of therapeutic touch and qigong therapy. *Journal of Complementary and Alternative Medicine,* 3 (2), 109-118.

Wirth, D.P., Richardson, J.T. and Eidelman, W.S. (1996). Wound healing and complementary therapies: A review. *Journal of Complementary and Alternative Medicine,* 2 (4), 493-502.

Index

SPECIAL 25%-OFF DISCOUNT!
Order a copy of this book with this form or online at:
http://www.haworthpressinc.com/store/product.asp?sku=4778

COMPLEMENTARY AND ALTERNATIVE MEDICINE
Clinic Design

_____in hardbound at $29.96 (regularly $39.95) (ISBN: 0-7890-1803-9)

_____in softbound at $18.71 (regularly $24.95) (ISBN: 0-7890-1804-7)

Or order online and use Code HEC25 in the shopping cart.

COST OF BOOKS_____

OUTSIDE US/CANADA/
MEXICO: ADD 20%_____

POSTAGE & HANDLING_____
*(US: $5.00 for first book & $2.00
for each additional book)
Outside US: $6.00 for first book
& $2.00 for each additional book)*

SUBTOTAL_____

IN CANADA: ADD 7% GST_____

STATE TAX_____
*(NY, OH & MN residents, please
add appropriate local sales tax)*

FINAL TOTAL_____
*(If paying in Canadian funds,
convert using the current
exchange rate, UNESCO
coupons welcome)*

☐ **BILL ME LATER:** ($5 service charge will be added)
(Bill-me option is good on US/Canada/Mexico orders only;
not good to jobbers, wholesalers, or subscription agencies.)

☐ Check here if billing address is different from
shipping address and attach purchase order and
billing address information.

Signature_____

☐ **PAYMENT ENCLOSED: $**_____

☐ **PLEASE CHARGE TO MY CREDIT CARD.**

☐ Visa ☐ MasterCard ☐ AmEx ☐ Discover
☐ Diner's Club ☐ Eurocard ☐ JCB

Account # _____

Exp. Date_____

Signature_____

Prices in US dollars and subject to change without notice.

NAME_____

INSTITUTION_____

ADDRESS_____

CITY_____

STATE/ZIP_____

COUNTRY_____ COUNTY (NY residents only)_____

TEL_____ FAX_____

E-MAIL_____

May we use your e-mail address for confirmations and other types of information? ☐ Yes ☐ No
We appreciate receiving your e-mail address and fax number. Haworth would like to e-mail or fax special
discount offers to you, as a preferred customer. **We will never share, rent, or exchange your e-mail address
or fax number.** We regard such actions as an invasion of your privacy.

Order From Your Local Bookstore or Directly From
The Haworth Press, Inc.
10 Alice Street, Binghamton, New York 13904-1580 • USA
TELEPHONE: 1-800-HAWORTH (1-800-429-6784) / Outside US/Canada: (607) 722-5857
FAX: 1-800-895-0582 / Outside US/Canada: (607) 722-6362
E-mail to: getinfo@haworthpressinc.com
PLEASE PHOTOCOPY THIS FORM FOR YOUR PERSONAL USE.
http://www.HaworthPress.com   BOF02